AOSpine Masters Series

Adult Spinal Deformities

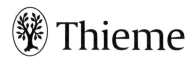

AOSpine Masters Series

Adult Spinal Deformities

Series Editor:
Luiz Roberto Vialle, MD, PhD
Professor of Orthopedics, School of Medicine
Catholic University of Parana State
Spine Unit
Curitiba, Brazil

Guest Editors:
Lawrence G. Lenke, MD
Jerome J. Gilden Distinguished Professor
Orthopaedic Surgery
Professor, Neurological Surgery
Chief of Spinal Surgery
Director of the Advanced Deformity Fellowship
Washington University School of Medicine
St. Louis, Missouri

Kenneth M.C. Cheung, MBBS(UK), MD (HK), FRCS, FHKCOS, FHKAM(Orth)
Head, Department of Orthopaedics & Traumatology
Jessie Ho Professor in Spine Surgery
The University of Hong Kong
Queen Mary Hospital
Pokfulam, Hong Kong

With 92 figures

Thieme
New York • Stuttgart • Delhi • Rio de Janeiro

Thieme Medical Publishers, Inc.
333 Seventh Ave.
New York, NY 10001

Executive Editor: William Lamsback
Managing Editor: Sarah Landis
Director, Editorial Services: Mary Jo Casey
Editorial Assistant: Haley Paskalides
Production Editor: Barbara A. Chernow
International Production Director: Andreas Schabert
Vice President, Editorial and E-Product Development: Vera Spillner
International Marketing Director: Fiona Henderson
International Sales Director: Louisa Turrell
Director of Sales, North America: Mike Roseman
Senior Vice President and Chief Operating Officer: Sarah Vanderbilt
President: Brian D. Scanlan
Compositor: Carol Pierson, Chernow Editorial Services, Inc.

Library of Congress Cataloging-in-Publication Data

AOSpine masters series. v. 4, Adult spinal deformities / editors, Luiz Roberto Vialle, Lawrence G. Lenke,
Kenneth M.C. Cheung.
    p. ; cm.
  Adult spinal deformities
  Includes bibliographical references and index.
  ISBN 978-1-62623-100-9 (alk. paper) – ISBN 978-1-62623-101-6 (eISBN)
  I. Vialle, Luiz Roberto, editor. II. Lenke, Lawrence, 1960– , editor. III. Cheung, Kenneth M. C., editor.
IV. Title: Adult spinal deformities.
  [DNLM: 1. Spinal Diseases—surgery. 2. Orthopedic Procedures—methods. 3. Spine—surgery. WE 725]
  RD768
  617.4'71—dc23   2015001979

Printed in China by Everbest Printing Ltd.
5 4 3 2 1
ISBN 978-1-62623-100-9

Also available as an e-book:
eISBN 978-1-62623-101-6

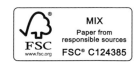

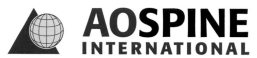

AOSpine Masters Series

Luiz Roberto Vialle, MD, PhD
Series Editor

Contents

Series Preface

Spine care is advancing at a rapid pace. The challenge for today's spine care professional is to quickly synthesize the best available evidence and expert opinion in the management of spine pathologies. The AOSpine Masters Series provides just that—each volume in the series delivers pathology-focused expert opinion on procedures, diagnosis, clinical wisdom, and pitfalls, and highlights today's top research papers.

To bring the value of its masters level educational courses and academic congresses to a wider audience, AOSpine has assembled internationally recognized spine pathology leaders to develop volumes in this Masters Series as a vehicle for sharing their experiences and expertise and providing links to the literature. Each volume focuses on a current compelling and sometimes controversial topic in spine care.

The unique and efficient format of the Masters Series volumes quickly focuses the attention of the reader on the core information critical to understanding the topic, while encouraging the reader to look further into the recommended literature.

Through this approach, AOSpine is advancing spine care worldwide.

Luiz Roberto Vialle, MD, PhD

Guest Editors' Preface

Adult spinal deformity (ASD) is a clinical problem of increasing prevalence, and thus physicians and patients worldwide are aware of it. With increasing longevity, the normal degeneration of the spine may lead to various ASD problems such as lumbar degenerative scoliosis with or without accompanying spinal kyphosis. In addition, ASD includes a spectrum of preexistent childhood deformities, such as scoliosis or kyphosis, that slowly progress to symptomatic stages over adulthood. Clinical manifestations may include progressive deformity, potential spinal imbalance, and spinal stenosis, with resultant axial or lower extremity symptomatology. Health-related quality-of-life assessments often demonstrate severe adverse effects of ASD that can interfere with many aspects of physical, emotional, and psychological well-being. When clinical and radiographic scenarios warrant, surgical intervention, ranging from simple decompressions to complex total spine reconstructions, should be considered in appropriate patients.

We have assembled a global panel of specialists to share with us their experience in the management of ASD, from evaluation to treatment, and including such issues as instrumentation and surgical techniques, as well as preventing and managing complications. Thorough patient evaluation, both medical and surgical, is warranted, with patient selection for indicated surgical intervention one of the main keys to a successful outcome. Pertinent issues, such as bone density evaluation and preoperative optimization, must be addressed with the use of intraoperative adjuvants to ensure stable internal fixation to the spinal column in patients requiring stabilization with or without realignment. For patients with progressive deformity producing segmental, regional, or global malalignment, various corrective strategies are discussed to safely realign the spinal column using various forms of spinal osteotomies with adjuvant spinal instrumentation to secure the spinal segments in their realigned position. Spinal fixation techniques are especially challenging when instrumenting the sacropelvic unit in long constructs. The various forms of osteotomies utilized range from simple facet excisions to extremely complex three-column osteotomies such as pedicle subtraction and vertebral column resection techniques that are occasionally required for patients with severe deformity with accompanying imbalance. Ensuring neurologic safety during ASD surgery is paramount, because these operations have an early neurologic complication rate that is not insignificant and can lead to permanent deficits. All of these essential preoperative and intraoperative factors are discussed in detail.

Even with initial surgical success, the long-term success of surgery for ASD is controversial. Various factors, such as wound infections, pseudarthrosis, and adjacent segment pathology, the most common being proximal junctional kyphosis (PJK), can lead to deterioration of the clinical outcomes over time. The durability of clinical outcome measures for these patients is an important focus along with the financial implications for treating ASD patients. Thus, as in all areas of medicine, the value proposition of treating ASD patients, both with nonoperative and operative procedures, must be ascertained to justify the wide spectrum of interventions available. As in all areas of surgery, selecting the appropriate patient and performing the least aggressive surgery to solve the clinical problem while ensuring long-term success is the optimal approach.

We hope this book will help spine surgeons from around the world navigate the often controversial and complicated clinical issues involved in the management of ASD patients, so that the outcome can be maximized and the complications minimized.

Lawrence G. Lenke, MD
Kenneth M.C. Cheung, MBBS(UK), MD (HK),
FRCS, FHKCOS, FHKAM(Orth)

Contributors

Yuichiro Abe, MD, PhD
Attending Spine Surgeon
Department of Orthopaedic Surgery
Eniwa Hospital
Eniwa, Japan

Ahmet Alanay, MD
Professor
Department of Orthopedics and
    Traumatology
Faculty of Medicine
Acibadem University
Istanbul, Turkey

Sigurd Berven, MD
Professor in Residence
Director of Spine Fellowship and Resident
    Education Program
Department of Orthopaedic Surgery
University of California–San Francisco
San Francisco, California

Joseph S. Butler, PhD, FRCS (Tr&Orth)
Clinical Fellow
Spinal Deformity Unit
Royal National Orthopaedic Hospital
Stanmore, Middlesex, United Kingdom

**Jason P.Y. Cheung, MBBS, MMedSc, FHKCOS,
    FHKAM(Orth), FRCSEd(Orth)**
Clinical Assistant Professor
Department of Orthopaedics & Traumatology
The University of Hong Kong
Queen Mary Hospital
Pokfulam, Hong Kong

**Kenneth M.C. Cheung, MBBS(UK), MD (HK),
    FRCS, FHKCOS, FHKAM(Orth)**
Head, Department of Orthopaedics &
    Traumatology
Jessie Ho Professor in Spine Surgery
The University of Hong Kong
Queen Mary Hospital
Pokfulam, Hong Kong

Simon A. Harris, MA, MB, BChir, FRCSC
Fellow
Department of Orthopedics
Toronto Western Hospital, University of
    Toronto
Toronto, Ontario, Canada

Manabu Ito, MD, PhD
Director
Center for Spine and Spinal Cord Disorders
National Hospital Organization Hokkaido
    Medical Center
Sapporo, Japan

Sravisht Iyer, MD
Orthopaedic Surgery Resident
Hospital for Special Surgery
New York, New York

Kristen E. Jones, MD
Fellow
Departments of Orthopaedic Surgery and
   Neurosurgery
University of Minnesota
Mineapolis, Minnesota

Daniel G. Kang , MD
Spine Surgery Fellow
Department of Orthopedic Surgery
Washington University
St. Louis, Missouri

Michael P. Kelly, MD, MSc
Assistant Professor of Orthopedic Surgery
Assistant Professor of Neurological Surgery
Department of Orthopedic Surgery
Washington University School of Medicine
Saint Louis, Missouri

Han Jo Kim, MD
Assistant Professor of Orthopaedic Surgery
Co-Director of Education
Spine Service
Hospital for Special Surgery
New York, New York

Ronald A. Lehman, Jr., MD
Professor of Orthopaedic Surgery
Professor of Neurological Surgery
Washington University School of Medicine
BJC Institute of Health
St. Louis, Missouri

Lawrence G. Lenke, MD
Jerome J. Gilden Distinguished Professor
Distinguished Professor of Orthopaedic Surgery
Professor of Neurological Surgery
Chief of Spinal Surgery
Director of the Advanced Deformity
   Fellowship
Washington University School of Medicine
St. Louis, Missouri

Stephen J. Lewis, MD, MSc, FRCSC
Associate Professor
University of Toronto
Department of Surgery
Division of Orthopaedics
Toronto Western Hospital for Sick
   Children
Toronto, Ontario, Canada

Robert A. Morgan, MD
Assistant Professor
Orthopaedic Surgeon
University of Minnesota
Minneapolis, Minnesota

David W. Polly, Jr., MD
Professor and Chief
Spine Service
University of Minnesota
Department of Orthopaedic Surgery
Minneapolis, Minnesota

Yong Qiu, MD
Professor and Director
Department of Spine Surgery
Nanjing Drum Tower Hospital
Medical School of Nanjing University
Nanjing, Jiangsu Province, China

Remel Alingalan Salmingo, PhD
Visiting Researcher
Biomedical Engineering
Technical University of Denmark (DTU)
Engineer
JJ X-Ray A/S
Technical University of Denmark (DTU)
   Scion
Kongens Lyngby, Denmark

Christopher I. Shaffrey, Sr., MD
John A. Jane Professor of Neurological
   Surgery
Professor of Orthopaedic Surgery
Department of Neurological Surgery
University of Virginia School of
   Medicine
Charlottesville, Virginia VA

Scott C. Wagner, MD
Instructor of Surgery
Division of Surgery
Department of Orthopaedics
Uniformed Services University of the Health
   Sciences
Walter Reed National Military Medical Center
Bethesda, Maryland

Robert Waldrop, MD
Fellow in Spine Surgery
Department of Orthopaedic Surgery
University of California–San Francisco
San Francisco, California

Caglar Yilgor, MD
Assistant Professor
Department of Orthopedics and
   Traumatology
Faculty of Medicine
Acibadem University
Istanbul, Turkey

1

Preoperative Evaluation and Optimization for Surgery

Scott C. Wagner, Daniel G. Kang, Ronald A. Lehman, Jr., and Lawrence G. Lenke

■ Introduction

Adult spinal deformity is an umbrella term encompassing various developmental, progressive, or degenerative conditions that contribute to an altered three dimensional structure of the human spine. There are three main types of adult spinal deformity: type 1, de novo, or primary degenerative scoliosis; type 2, untreated adolescent idiopathic scoliosis that has progressed into adulthood; and type 3, secondary scoliosis related to altered vertebral anatomy due to previous surgery, trauma, or metabolic bone disease.[1] A secondary form of adult scoliosis is iatrogenic imbalance caused by previous spinal surgery.[2] The most clinically important and most commonly encountered types of adult deformity are types 1 and 3.[1]

Structural curves that develop in adulthood (type 1) generally begin and then progress as the intervertebral disks degenerate with normal aging. As disk degeneration progresses, posterior element incompetence leads to axial rotation of the spinal motion segments, with permanent rotatory deformity in turn leading to ligamentous laxity and eventual lateral listhesis of the vertebral bodies.[3] Destruction of the diskoligamentous complex and ensuing degeneration of the facet joints leads to abnormal motion at each vertebral segment, subsequently causing reactive changes such as osteophytosis at the end plates, facet joint hypertrophy/cysts, and ligamentum flavum hypertrophy. In addi-

tion, the concavity of the major and fractional curve can cause foraminal narrowing, which is often further exacerbated by disk degeneration and loss of foraminal height (up/down foraminal stenosis). These changes cause narrowing of the spinal canal (central and lateral recess) and neural foramen,[1] and collectively contribute to the clinical symptoms of adult scoliosis or spinal deformity. Thus, understanding the complex pathomechanics and anatomy of this degenerative process is vital for spine surgeons considering performing deformity surgery. As the population ages and life expectancy increases, the prevalence of degenerative adult spinal deformity will continue to increase.[2] In fact, the impact on overall public health and disability of the United States population by adult degenerative scoliosis cannot be overstated, and there will likely be an increased number of these patients electing surgical correction of their deformity and treatment of their symptoms.[2,4]

■ Epidemiology

New-onset adult degenerative deformities are considered in the context of a population older than 40 years of age, without a prior history of adolescent idiopathic scoliosis (AIS). Adult scoliosis can be asymptomatic, and the incidence of spinal curves of less than 10 degrees may be as high as 64%.[5] In fact, 30% of elderly patients without a previous history of spinal deformity will develop new structural abnormalities, with men and women affected equally (in contrast to adolescent idiopathic scoliosis, in which girls are more commonly affected than boys).[3] Patients with progressive degenerative spinal deformities typically present in the sixth decade with various symptoms, frequently including a combination of back pain, radiculopathy, and neurogenic claudication.[3] Adult degenerative deformities tend to progress up to 6 degrees per year, averaging 3 degrees per year, if left untreated,[3] and radiographic parameters that predict a high risk for progression include a Cobb angle greater than 30 degrees, lateral olisthesis greater than 6 mm, and a large degree of apical rotation.[3] However, open surgical spinal deformity correction in adult patients is associated with a complication rate of up to 86%, including a 7.8% rate of early wound infection, and is typically associated with large amounts of intraoperative blood loss, deep wound infection, and pulmonary embolism.[4,6,7]

Therefore, thorough preoperative evaluation and optimization is absolutely paramount when considering surgical treatment of adult spinal deformity, because this patient population is often elderly, with multiple associated comorbidities, and at high risk for medical and surgical complications.[8] A multidisciplinary approach, including the primary care provider, an internist, an endocrinologist, a cardiologist, as well as the treating spine surgeon, should be undertaken in the perioperative evaluation process to minimize the potential medical risks and maximize the functional benefits.

▨ Clinical Evaluation

Initial Assessment

The initial assessment must include taking a comprehensive history and performing a thorough physical examination. A previous diagnosis of spinal deformity (e.g., adolescent idiopathic scoliosis, kyphosis, congenital deformity), a history of prior spine surgeries, as well as any previous imaging studies demonstrating progression of degenerative changes and deformity will provide clinical cues to appropriately guide the remainder of the workup. Patients typically present with a combination of various complaints, including upper or lower back pain, radiating lower extremity pain or weakness, paresthesias/numbness, neurogenic claudication, difficulty with gait or upright posture, and progression of their deformity. Changes in body habitus/posture (particularly changes in the fit of clothing), difficulty with gait or decreased walking distance tolerance, and changes in the use of assistive devices are elicited during the history-taking process. Back pain is the most common presenting symptom, and complaints of pain must be differentiated with regard to axial versus radicular symptoms. Isolated low back pain may represent paraspinal muscle fatigue or mechanical instability at the painful segment,[1] with increased pain severity often suggesting significant sagittal and coronal imbalance.[3] If radicular pain is present in addition to axial pain, duration/onset of symptoms, exacerbating activities, and laterality of the symptoms provide guidance for potential decompression.[1,3] Radicular extremity pain can be caused by an acute disk herniation, localized foraminal or lateral recess nerve root compression from osteophytes/spondylotic changes, foraminal compression on the concave side of the fractional curve, or traction on the convex side of the deformity, or may be related instead to single- or multilevel central stenosis. Neurologic deficits are less common in adult deformities, but when present are often related to segmental instability causing foraminal compression or congenital spinal stenosis, which is exacerbated by degenerative changes causing further central canal stenosis.[1] The operative approach should take into consideration the extent and type of decompression and fusion construct, if any, that is indicated based on the patient's symptomatology, as well as any recent changes or progression of symptoms.[1]

The clinical examination includes assessment of a shift in the trunk, and the relationship of the head to the pelvis in the coronal and sagittal plane is noted. Asymmetry of the shoulder or pelvic girdles provides useful information with regard to the severity of the deformity, as do pelvic obliquity and leg-length discrepancy. Other subtle clues to severity and progression of the deformity include skin creases around the trunk/abdomen and standing posture (e.g., pelvic retroversion, hip/knee flexion). Having the patient perform forward and lateral bending during the exam can provide important prognostic information, as the rigidity of the curve can affect the overall outcome of nonoperative and subsequent operative intervention. Hip and knee flexion contractures should also be assessed with the patient lying in the supine position on the examination table. Then, with the patient lying in the prone position on the table, the flexibility of the curve without gravity can be determined, and the patient's ability to tolerate the prone position and overall physical conditioning can be assessed. The patient's inability to turn prone independently may indicate significant deconditioning and that the patient is a high-risk surgical candidate). Neurovascular examination includes overall gait assessment, motor strength, deep tendon reflexes, sensation and cranial nerve function, as well as extremity pulse assessment.[3] The patient should also be examined for long tract signs, as myelopathy may be a component of severe thoracic deformity, as well as to ensure that the patient does not have concomitant cervical stenosis.

Radiographic Evaluation

Radiographic evaluation includes full-length standing anteroposterior and lateral radiographs of the spine, with the patient's knees and hips straight, as well as supine full-length films to provide information regarding any spontaneous deformity reduction with gravity forces removed. Cobb angle measurements and radiographic determination of spinopelvic imbalance provide critical information, as the degree of the curve and the extent of imbalance can necessitate discussion of operative intervention at the time of initial evaluation. For the purpose of preoperative planning, these measurements are imperative. Rotatory subluxation, the presence and location of osteophytosis, and any anteroposterior or lateral listhesis

are noted. Magnetic resonance imaging (MRI) is routinely obtained, particularly in the presence of radicular pain or neurologic symptoms, though it is not uncommon for these older patients to be unable to undergo an MRI for various reasons (e.g., presence of a pacemaker). Also, in the revision setting, previous spinal instrumentation may cause significant image artifact and difficulty in MRI interpretation. In such patients, computed tomography (CT) myelogram is obtained instead of MRI, and provides information regarding significant areas of stenosis. We also routinely obtain a CT scan in adult spinal deformity patients for preoperative planning, which enables evaluation of the extent of spondylotic changes and the levels/areas of autofusion, helps determine the feasibility and sizing of spinal fixation points, and, in the revision setting, helps analyze the location/size of any previous decompressions, the healing of previously fused regions, and the position of previous spinal instrumentation. In addition, at our institution, the CT scan is useful in patients with complex deformity (e.g., congenital/segmentation abnormalities, significant angular deformity, previous postsurgical changes) through the use of a three-dimensional acrylic model for preoperative planning, and can also be used intraoperatively to identify topographic landmarks and guide placement of instrumentation.

Provocative Testing

Selective nerve root/transforaminal corticosteroid injections can also be used to provide diagnostic information as well as a therapeutic effect.[1] We use selective nerve root/transforaminal injections in patients with a component of radicular/lower extremity pain to help determine the specific nerve root causing symptoms, provide temporary relief prior to surgical treatment, and ultimately to localize the levels in which decompression may result in symptom relief. However, the utility of selective nerve root/transforaminal injections remains unclear, as the lack of response to the injection may be attributable to the injection technique or to poor patient recall. We specifically ask the patient about the immediate relief of symptoms, within 5 to 10 minutes following the injection, as a criterion for a diagnostic injection (symptoms likely arising from that level of injection). In contrast, an injection causing relief hours or days later may be a function of the systemic anti-inflammatory effect following systemic absorption of the corticosteroid. Similarly, in our experience, epidural corticosteroid injections provide limited diagnostic information, as the corticosteroid medication distributes throughout multiple levels and is also absorbed systemically. However, we offer epidural corticosteroid injections for patients with significant central or lateral recess stenosis to potentially provide temporary relief of symptoms and improve physical function to enable preoperative optimization of fitness and mobility. We do not routinely use facet blocks or diskography for diagnostic assessment in the adult spinal deformity patient.[9] However, in patients with isolated axial back pain and arthritic facet changes on imaging studies, facet blocks may be utilized. Because the pain generator can be located at any point in the spine relative to the apex of the curve, facet blocks are performed sequentially at different levels to isolate specifically which motion segments are causing the pain, with subsequent relief of symptoms after injection/ablation.[1]

■ Nonoperative Management

A trial of nonoperative management is indicated for almost all patients presenting with adult spinal deformities, particularly curves of less than 30 degrees, less than 2 mm of listhesis, and if the constellation of symptoms is relatively minor. In contradistinction to the treatment algorithm of adolescent idiopathic scoliosis, there is no role for bracing in adult spinal deformity patients[3] because the progression of the curve is related to degenerative changes and mechanical instability, and not longitudinal growth of the axial skeleton. Therefore, the benefit of temporary pain relief is outweighed by the potential deconditioning of the paraspinal muscles and by skin complications resulting from brace treatment in this patient population.[3,10]

However, in rare cases in which the pain source cannot be adequately localized, thoracolumbar or thoracolumbosacral orthoses (TLO/TLSO) may be considered for temporary stabilization and pain relief.[1] Low-impact core strengthening programs and physical therapy are utilized to improve patient reserves as well as to stabilize the surrounding musculature to provide improved support to the spinal column.[3] Nonsteroidal anti-inflammatory drugs (NSAIDs) are used to provide relief of axial and, occasionally, radicular pain and neurogenic claudication. We do not routinely provide narcotic pain medications for nonoperative treatment, and pain management specialists are consulted to provide multimodal therapy with optimization of nonnarcotic pain medications (e.g., gabapentin, pregabalin), although sometimes short periods of narcotics or pain medications may be necessary. Also if operative treatment is decided, we encourage reduction or complete discontinuation of any narcotic pain medications to avoid difficult pain management in the postoperative period.

■ Surgical Indications

Indications for surgery in these patients include failure of nonoperative pain management with significantly diminished quality of life/function, or progression of deformity/imbalance, with correlation between radiographic and clinical findings. As previously mentioned, lumbar curves greater than 30 degrees or with 6 mm of listhesis in any plane are considered for surgery because the deformity is at high risk for progression. Also, patients with annual deformity progression greater than 10 degrees or with increasing listhesis (lateral, anterior, or posterior) greater than 3 mm, and whose symptoms are progressively worsening, are offered surgical stabilization. Ultimately, the decision to proceed with surgical management is predicated on several major factors, including the patient's symptomatology, age, general medical health, and the patient's expectations with regard to the outcome of such a significant procedure.[1] If surgical options are to be pursued, medical optimization of the patient and detailed preoperative surgical planning are absolutely critical to promote the success of the treatment plan.

■ Optimization for Surgery

As previously mentioned, the presenting age of patients with adult spinal deformities is typically between 60 and 70 years, and systemic medical comorbidities are common.[1,3] Diabetes and cardiac and vascular disease can significantly impact the surgical outcome, particularly for a large reconstructive procedure, given the potential for considerable intraoperative blood loss and overall surgical time.[1,3] Postoperatively, elderly patients also require longer rehabilitation, given their decreased cardiopulmonary reserves.[1] Therefore, consultation with the anesthesiologist and the patient's primary care provider is recommended to pursue an interdisciplinary approach for stratifying the patient's perioperative medical risks and optimizing medical comorbidities prior to proceeding with surgery.

Halpin et al[11] and Sugrue et al[12] described their high-risk protocol for patients undergoing major spinal surgery: patients are considered high risk if the surgeon anticipates longer than 6 hours of operative time, more than six vertebral levels will be included, or that the procedure will be staged, or if the patient presents with significant medical comorbidities. In these authors' protocols, all high-risk patients are evaluated by a hospitalist and anesthesiologist, and various parameters are evaluated and optimized, including nutritional status, pulmonary status, cardiac and renal function, and hepatic function.[11,12] The case is then discussed at a conference for high-risk spine procedures that is attended by all managing providers before operative clearance is granted.[11] At our institution, the use of similar goal-directed, evidence-based protocols to coordinate the care of complex patients has improved outcomes and overall patient satisfaction postoperatively.[12]

Nutritional status of the adult spinal deformity patient should be assessed preoperatively. This evaluation is typically accomplished by measuring serum albumin, prealbumin, total protein, and transferrin, which provide information regarding patient protein reserves.[13] Patients with albumin levels less than 3.5 g per deciliter have been shown to have a significantly higher risk of complications and mortality.[14] Prealbumin levels below 11 mg per deciliter require nutritional support, and because these levels are not affected by hydration status, prealbumin is the recommended measurement tool for assessing nutritional status.[14] Any insufficiency in the nutritional state identified preoperatively should be corrected prior to surgery, consulting with a nutritionist if necessary. The duration of nutritional support is dependent on the severity of the malnourished state and the patient's general health, but generally is 6 to 12 weeks in order to attain appropriate nutritional optimization, although some patients may require a longer period. Postoperative nutrition is an important aspect for all patients following spinal deformity surgery, particularly with complex spinal reconstructive procedures that entail significant metabolic demand. There is often a balance in timing for the start of nutrition by mouth and return of bowel function (i.e., bowel sound, flatus, and bowel movement). Starting an oral diet too early may result in ileus or obstruction, which can significantly increase the patient's pain and limit early rehabilitation efforts, whereas unnecessarily delaying the start of nutrition may fail to meet metabolic requirements to optimize healing and rehabilitation in the postoperative period. Therefore, in certain cases, particularly following complex spinal reconstructive procedures, we attempt placement of a small bowel feeding tube (SBFT) on postoperative day 1, with the goal to begin tube feeds by postoperative day 2. If there is difficulty in placing the SBFT distal to the pylorus, we begin parenteral nutrition support through central access. We continue small bowel tube feeds or parenteral nutrition support until the patient is tolerating adequate nutrition by mouth.

Perioperative blood management is an aspect of adult spinal deformity surgery that requires particular attention. Low preoperative hemoglobin concentration and increased number of levels fused have been shown to be significant risk factors for allogeneic blood transfusion at the time of surgery.[15] The risks associated with transfusion are myriad, and include benign febrile reaction, infectious disease transmission, and anaphylaxis. Therefore, efforts to reduce the potential need for transfusion should be undertaken preoperatively. In the absence of any contraindications, we recommend that patients with adult spinal deformity take iron supplements for 2 to 4 weeks prior to surgery.[14] There is evidence to suggest that preoperative recombinant human erythropoietin (rhEPO) administration in the preoperative period can reduce the transfusion rate without increasing complications.[16] However, at our institution this is not a common practice given the significant expense of rhEPO, and, in our experience, its limited effectiveness in the adult spinal deformity patient. We typically use other perioperative adjunctive measures and blood management strategies, which includes the use of intravenous antifibrinolytics (e.g., tranexamic acid), cell saver, and topical hemostatic agents (e.g., Surgiflo, thrombin), as well as paying meticulous attention to hemostasis throughout the procedure (including packing off segments with rolled surgical sponges to reduce blood loss when attention is focused on decompressing or instrumenting more cephalad or caudad spinal levels).

Open anterior surgical deformity correction for severe spinal deformity has been shown to have detrimental effects on postoperative pulmonary function, particularly in older adult patients or patients with preexisting lung disease.[17,18] Although pulmonary function testing is not routinely performed preoperatively, we typically evaluate patients with pulmonary symptoms, difficulty with or poor endurance with daily activity and ambulation, or complex or severe thoracic deformity (often with planned three-column osteotomy). We use pulmonary function testing in these patients to stratify the risk of potential postoperative pulmonary complications, and we obtain a pulmonary specialist consultation for perioperative optimization. Also, preoperative smoking cessation is imperative for at least 8 weeks prior to surgery.

Typically, major deformity correction and fusion has been accomplished via combined anterior/posterior approaches; the anterior release with fusion is achieved via a thoracotomy or thoracoabdominal approach, followed by posterior instrumentation, which provides improved fusion rates and better overall correction.[19] However, it is postulated that disruption of the thoracic cage during the anterior approach leads to injury to the respiratory mechanism.[18] Because of this theory, there has been interest in posterior-only management of severe deformities (e.g., via three-column osteotomies such as pedicle substraction osteotomy [PSO] or vertebral column resection [VCR]) and in the theoretical benefits of obviating the anterior approach on pulmonary function. There is some evidence that posterior-only surgery can achieve similar postoperative radiographic outcomes[19]; however, patients with such severe deformities often present with chronic restrictive lung disease, with minimal potential for improvement in lung function despite correction of the thoracic deformity, and a recent study found that, in adult patients, utilization of VCR for severe deformity correction did not improve postoperative pulmonary function.[18] Preoperative pulmonary function testing, therefore, may be worthwhile in patients with significant thoracic deformities and baseline pulmonary disease to establish potential reserves. Thus, it is important to counsel older patients with more severe deformities that despite the correction afforded by the surgery, which may require extensive osteotomies, pulmonary function may not improve significantly postoperatively.[18]

Hypovitaminosis D, although extremely common, is often missed in the preoperative setting, despite the potentially serious complications arising from this deficiency. It is estimated that more than half of all general medicine inpatients are deficient in vitamin D, though the prevalence in patients undergoing spine surgery remains largely unexplored.[20] A recent study from a single institution found an overall vitamin D deficiency rate of 57% in patients undergoing spinal surgery of any kind, and the rate for patients with diagnosed spinal deformity was 18%; this relatively low prevalence is likely attributable to an increased rate of vitamin D supplementation in this cohort.[20] It is thus important to consider this diagnosis and recommend adequate vitamin D intake for patients with diagnosed spinal deformity, especially preoperatively, as calcium metabolism is extremely important in the prevention of osteoporosis.

Along with hypovitaminosis D, osteoporosis is also very common in this patient population. The management of this serious disease requires the cooperation of a multidisciplinary team. Postmenopausal women are at a high risk for development and progression of osteoporosis, which can lead to fragility fractures and increased mortality; however, older men may also present with osteoporosis, and any clinical suspicion should prompt an initial workup. The World Health Organization (WHO) recommends that all peri- and postmenopausal women undergo screening for low bone mineral density (BMD),[21] and dual-energy X-ray absorptiometry (DEXA) is the gold standard for assessment of BMD. We obtain DEXA BMD measurements of the lumbar spine and hips for all preoperative patients, regardless of age or gender, to identify osteoporotic patients who may require optimization/treatment with consultation of an endocrinologist or primary care provider prior to surgery. Postmenopausal women diagnosed with osteoporosis should also receive 1,500 mg calcium and 400 IU vitamin D daily. There also exist medical modalities for optimization of BMD, including bisphosphonates, parathyroid hormone (teriparatide), estrogen modulators or hormone replacement, and calcitonin. The use of these medications should be monitored in consultation with the patient's endocrinologist or primary care provider. Identifying patients with osteoporosis prior to surgery facilitates treatment and optimization of their BMD, and can improve surgical outcomes by optimizing the fixation strength of the surgical instrumentation and ultimately improve bone healing/fusion.

Cardiopulmonary, nutritional, and bone-quality assessments are vital in this patient population. Comorbidities are intuitively more common in the adult deformity population when compared with the adolescent idiopathic scoliosis population, and the presence and severity of these comorbidities guide the initial management of the deformity. Although there has been some evidence that osteopenia and osteoporosis do not play a significant role in the progression of adult spinal deformity,[3] in patients electing to proceed with surgical correction of scoliosis the presence of osteoporosis can affect the ability to obtain purchase in the bony spine. In patients over 50 years of age undergoing spine surgery of any type, the incidence of osteoporosis has been reported to be 14.5% for men and 51.3% for women.[22] Indeed, osteoporosis is associated with reported fusion rates as low as 56%, as well as iatrogenic instability and fracture following surgery.[23] Surveys have found that most orthopedic spine surgeons feel uncomfortable managing the treatment of osteoporosis after it has been diagnosed[24]; therefore, prompt referral to primary care providers or endocrine specialists for partial or complete management of osteoporosis prior to any planned surgical procedure is recommended.

Lastly, psychosocial factors must be considered. Mental health issues are common in the older adult population, and the presence of depression, anxiety, psychosis, or other premorbid psychological conditions can adversely affect surgical outcomes and patient perception of surgical success.[11] These factors can be managed by effectively utilizing a team of social workers or case managers and psychiatric support, and should not be overlooked prior to undertaking major spinal deformity surgery.

■ Preventing Complications

Medical complications surrounding adult spinal deformity surgery can range from mild to extremely severe, with an overall complication rate ranging from 40 to 86% in patients undergoing deformity surgery.[25] Thorough attention to the preoperative medical optimization process can reduce the incidence of postoperative complications, and strategies to minimize such complications should be judiciously employed. The most common minor complication in the postoperative period is urinary tract infection (UTI), with a reported rate of 9%.[25] UTIs can be prevented pre- and intraoperatively by appropriate sterile technique during insertion of the catheter, unrestricted catheter drainage, early removal, and, in some instances, instillation of benign bacteria in the urinary tract.[25] Pulmonary abnormalities, including atelectasis and pneumonia, are also very common in this population. These complications can be prevented in the preoperative setting via smoking cessation at least 8 weeks prior to surgery, as noted above, as well as appropriate use of bronchodilators or pulmonary rehabilitation protocols.[25] Of course, many other intra- and postoperative strategies exist to minimize the numerous complications that may occur, but these are beyond the scope of this chapter.

■ Preoperative Planning

Levels of Treatment

Six levels of operative treatment were described by Silva and Lenke[3] in 2010: I, decompression alone; II, decompression and limited instrumented posterior spinal fusion; III, decompression and lumbar curve instrumented fusion; IV, decompression with anterior and posterior spinal instrumented fusion; V, thoracic instrumentation and fusion extension; and VI, inclusion of osteotomies for specific deformities. Each level represents a unique approach to surgical management of adult spinal deformity, predicated on the constellation of symptoms reported by the patient, and designed to provide independent symptom management. For patients with neurogenic claudication alone secondary to central canal stenosis, level I treatment, which entails limited decompression, is appropriate. These patients often present with minimal back pain, and radiographic analysis may reveal small osteophytes with less than 2 mm of subluxation. Additionally, these patients should have no cosmetic or major deformity complaints, and the coronal and sagittal balance must be within reason, as isolated central decompression in the presence of curves greater than 30 degrees (or with kyphosis) can

lead to worsening of the deformity.[3] A relatively large series found that coronal imbalance greater than 4 cm correlated with decreased overall patient-related outcome scores on the Scoliosis Research Society-22 (SRS-22) scale and the Oswestry Disability Index (ODI),[26] and thus these parameters are extremely important in the surgical decision-making process. However, for the relatively well-balanced patient with more than 2 mm of subluxation, the addition of posterior instrumentation at the level of the decompression improves stability and constitutes level II of treatment. If such patients also have complaints of significant lumbar pain associated with the lumbar deformity greater than 30 degrees, but maintain global sagittal and coronal alignment, the entire lumbar curve must be included in the instrumented region, which constitutes level III of treatment.[3] Transforaminal lumbar interbody fusion (TLIF) may also be utilized as an adjunct when fusing to the sacrum to improve fixation and fusion at the transitional lumbosacral junction.[3]

Loss of lumbar lordosis, often associated with flat-back syndrome in adult deformity patients, is often managed via an anterior fusion approach. Utilizing anterior fusion in addition to posterior fixation constitutes level IV and provides both load sharing to reduce posterior strain and additional cephalocaudad foraminal decompression.[3] In addition to the aforementioned criteria, patients with additional sagittal imbalance can be managed by expanding the fusion proximal to the thoracolumbar junction, which constitutes level V of treatment.[3] It is also important that anterior osteophytes be minimal, and significant thoracic kyphosis contraindicates this treatment approach.[3] Once significant sagittal or coronal imbalance has developed, spinal fusion without adjustment of global alignment will be insufficient to control symptoms. A recent retrospective study examining the role of preoperative coronal and sagittal balance found that postoperative correction of sagittal balance was the strongest predictor of clinical outcomes, whereas another study has suggested that severe preoperative coronal imbalance predicts worse functional recovery.[7,26] Historically, patients with severe, rigid spinal deformities have been managed with combined anterior/posterior approaches; however, there has been increased interest in the use of complex three-column osteotomies to enable an all posterior approach, however interest in the use of complex three-column osteotomies to enable an all posterior approach; the use of these osteotomies constitutes Level VI of surgical management. These complex three-column osteotomies require highly experienced surgeons and a specialized operating room team to ensure optimal outcomes and the highest level of safety, and even with this expertise there is still a 30 to 40% rate of complications following these procedures.[17]

■ Chapter Summary

Patients with adult spinal deformity represent some of the most complex surgical candidates in the population, and estimates suggest that the number of patients electing to undergo surgical correction will continue to increase. Adult scoliosis comprises a diverse spectrum of disease, with multiple potential etiologies and natural histories, and as such there is no one single approach to management that can be applied to all adult deformity patients. Radiographic, clinical, and subjective findings must be assessed preoperatively by a multidisciplinary team. Because these patients typically present after the sixth decade of life, with multiple associated medical comorbidities, the spine surgeon must be aware of the potential for significant risk exposure in the perioperative setting. A multidisciplinary approach to preoperative evaluation must be employed, and the patient's primary care provider, internist, endocrinologist, and cardiologist should be actively engaged in determining if the patient is appropriate for surgery and in preparing the patient for the procedure. If the patient is not currently being evaluated for major medical conditions common to this population, such as restrictive lung disease or osteoporosis, the spine surgeon may be the first provider to initiate assessment and recommend treatment. The complexity of the three-dimensional pathoanatomy and associated biomechanics that can significantly affect postoperative outcomes must be understood and respected, and the preoperative evaluation and optimization for surgery process must be tailored to each individual patient. With appropriate patient selection, understanding of all treatment options and decision algorithms, as well as understanding the importance of a team approach to perioperative medical management, spine surgeons can expect good results for their patients undergoing surgical treatment for adult spinal deformity.

Pearls

- ◆ Back pain is the most common complaint in adult spinal deformity patients.
- ◆ If claudication symptoms are present in addition to axial pain complaints, laterality of the pain provides guidance for potential decompression and likely instrumented fusion.
- ◆ The rigidity of the curve can be assessed both clinically and radiographically, and affects overall outcomes of nonoperative and subsequent operative intervention.
- ◆ Full-length standing anteroposterior and lateral radiographs of the spine are essential, and supine full-length films provide information regarding any spontaneous deformity reduction related to gravity.
- ◆ Indications for surgery in these patients include failure of nonoperative pain management, as well as correlation between radiographic and clinical findings.
- ◆ Consultation with the anesthesiologist and the patient's primary care provider is recommended to ensure an multidisciplinary approach for stratifying the patient's perioperative medical risks and optimizing medical comorbidities prior to proceeding with surgery
- ◆ Preoperative pulmonary function should be evaluated, as increased impairment or minimal improvement in pulmonary function can be expected postoperatively, and patients should be informed about this matter.
- ◆ Hypovitaminosis D and osteoporosis are extremely common in this patient population, and, given the significant detrimental effect on fusion rates and potentially overall clinical outcomes, should be managed in consultation with an endocrinologist.
- ◆ Operative candidates can be classified based on severity and type of their symptoms, as well as preoperative radiographic findings.
- ◆ Consideration should be given to posterior-only deformity correction techniques, which may reduce morbidity associated with the anterior thoracotomy or thoracoabdominal approaches.

Pitfalls

- Bracing is not routinely utilized in adult spinal deformity patients and may result in deconditioning and skin complications.
- Failure to identify and evaluate osteoporosis and subsequently failing to optimize BMD may result in suboptimal fixation and construct/fusion failure.
- Patients may flex their knees and hips, with subsequent pelvic retroversion, to compensate for fixed sagittal imbalance, and the surgeon should ensure that radiographs are obtained without these compensatory mechanisms.
- Narcotic pain medications should not be routinely prescribed preoperatively, and patients with significant narcotic pain medication use preopera-

tively should be weaned to optimize postoperative pain management.
- Failure to identify preoperative nutritional deficiency may result in poor wound healing, difficulty with rehabilitation, and prolonged fusion healing.
- Complex three-column osteotomies require highly experienced spine surgeons and a specialized operating room team to ensure optimal outcomes and the highest level of safety. Therefore, the spine surgeon should always consider every other option or technique to obtain realignment and optimize balance (e.g., positioning, posterior soft tissue/ligament releases, facetectomies, posterior column osteotomy) rather than use a three-column osteotomy.

References

Five Must-Read References

1. Aebi M. The adult scoliosis. Eur Spine J 2005;14:925–948
2. Mesfin A, Lenke LG, Bridwell KH, et al. Does preoperative narcotic use adversely affect outcomes and complications after spinal deformity surgery? A comparison of nonnarcotic- with narcotic-using groups. Spine J 2014;14:2819–2825
3. Silva FE, Lenke LG. Adult degenerative scoliosis: evaluation and management. Neurosurg Focus 2010; 28:E1
4. Mummaneni PV, Shaffrey CI, Lenke LG, et al; Minimally Invasive Surgery Section of the International Spine Study Group. The minimally invasive spinal deformity surgery algorithm: a reproducible rational framework for decision making in minimally invasive spinal deformity surgery. Neurosurg Focus 2014;36:E6
5. Schwab F, Dubey A, Gamez L, et al. Adult scoliosis: prevalence, SF-36, and nutritional parameters in an elderly volunteer population. Spine 2005;30:1082–1085
6. Schwab FJ, Hawkinson N, Lafage V, et al; International Spine Study Group. Risk factors for major perioperative complications in adult spinal deformity surgery: a multi-center review of 953 consecutive patients. Eur Spine J 2012;21:2603–2610
7. Daubs MD, Lenke LG, Bridwell KH, et al. Does correction of preoperative coronal imbalance make a difference in outcomes of adult patients with deformity? Spine 2013;38:476–483
8. Acosta FL Jr, McClendon J Jr, O'Shaughnessy BA, et al. Morbidity and mortality after spinal deformity surgery in patients 75 years and older: complications and predictive factors. J Neurosurg Spine 2011;15:667–674
9. Grubb SA, Lipscomb HJ, Suh PB. Results of surgical treatment of painful adult scoliosis. Spine 1994;19:1619–1627
10. van Dam BE. Nonoperative treatment of adult scoliosis. Orthop Clin North Am 1988;19:347–351
11. Halpin RJ, Sugrue PA, Gould RW, et al. Standardizing care for high-risk patients in spine surgery: the Northwestern high-risk spine protocol. Spine 2010;35:2232–2238
12. Sugrue PA, Halpin RJ, Koski TR. Treatment algorithms and protocol practice in high-risk spine surgery. Neurosurg Clin N Am 2013;24:219–230
13. Klein JD, Hey LA, Yu CS, et al. Perioperative nutrition and postoperative complications in patients undergoing spinal surgery. Spine 1996;21:2676–2682
14. Kelly MP, Hu SS. Nutrition and pain management in the adult spinal deformity patient. Scoliosis Research Society e-text. http://etext.srs.org/. Accessed August 30, 2014
15. Nuttall GA, Horlocker TT, Santrach PJ, Oliver WC Jr, Dekutoski MB, Bryant S. Predictors of blood transfusions in spinal instrumentation and fusion surgery. Spine 2000;25:596–601
16. Shapiro GS, Boachie-Adjei O, Dhawlikar SH, Maier LS. The use of Epoetin alfa in complex spine deformity surgery. Spine 2002;27:2067–2071
17. Auerbach JD, Lenke LG, Bridwell KH, et al. Major complications and comparison between 3-column osteotomy techniques in 105 consecutive spinal deformity procedures. Spine 2012;37:1198–1210
18. Bumpass DB, Lenke LG, Bridwell KH, et al. Pulmonary function improvement after vertebral column resection for severe spinal deformity. Spine 2014;39:587–595

19. Good CR, Lenke LG, Bridwell KH, et al. Can posterior-only surgery provide similar radiographic and clinical results as combined anterior (thoracotomy/thoraco-abdominal)/posterior approaches for adult scoliosis? Spine 2010;35:210–218

20. Stoker GE, Buchowski JM, Bridwell KH, Lenke LG, Riew KD, Zebala LP. Preoperative vitamin D status of adults undergoing surgical spinal fusion. Spine 2013; 38:507–515

21. Lane JM, Nydick M. Osteoporosis: current modes of prevention and treatment. J Am Acad Orthop Surg 1999;7:19–31

22. Chin DK, Park JY, Yoon YS, et al. Prevalence of osteoporosis in patients requiring spine surgery: incidence and significance of osteoporosis in spine disease. Osteoporos Int 2007;18:1219–1224

23. Park SB, Chung CK. Strategies of spinal fusion on osteoporotic spine. J Korean Neurosurg Soc 2011;49: 317–322

24. Dipaola CP, Bible JE, Biswas D, Dipaola M, Grauer JN, Rechtine GR. Survey of spine surgeons on attitudes regarding osteoporosis and osteomalacia screening and treatment for fractures, fusion surgery, and pseudoarthrosis. Spine J 2009;9:537–544

25. Baron EM, Albert TJ. Medical complications of surgical treatment of adult spinal deformity and how to avoid them. Spine 2006;31(19, Suppl):S106–S118

26. Glassman SD, Berven S, Bridwell K, Horton W, Dimar JR. Correlation of radiographic parameters and clinical symptoms in adult scoliosis. Spine 2005;30:682–688.

2

Decision Making in Adult Deformity Surgery: Decompression Versus Short or Long Fusion

Kenneth M.C. Cheung and Jason P.Y. Cheung

▇ Introduction

Degenerative scoliosis most commonly affects the lumbar spine in the elderly. It occurs as a result of facet and disk degeneration, leading to increased loads and resulting deformity. The prevalence of adult scoliosis in the elderly population may be as high as 68%,[1] and this number will only increase as people live longer and want to maintain their activity levels. Untreated scoliosis can lead to pain, spinal osteoarthritis, worsening deformity, spinal stenosis with radiculopathy, coronal and sagittal imbalance, associated muscle fatigue, and psychological effects from poor cosmesis and reduced mobility.

The management of adult deformity is controversial, with a lack of high-quality evidence to guide treatment, such as determining the best candidates for conservative versus surgical treatment, and the best surgical procedures for specific clinical scenarios. Nevertheless, patients tend to present with back or leg pain, and concerns about deformity progression need to be addressed. Thus, an understanding of the possible causes is important before appropriate recommendations for treatment can be made.

▇ Diagnosis of Back Pain

One of the most common presenting yet difficult-to-discern complaints of degenerative

scoliosis is back pain. The pain may be static or mechanical, localized or regional, or associated with buttock or leg pain, and there may even be neurologic symptoms. It is important to elicit a thorough history documenting the pain's severity, its aggravating and relieving factors, and its functional limitations that affect work or recreation or reduce the patient's ability to walk distances. This information helps elucidate the cause of the pain, and thus helps in determining the appropriate treatment.

Axial back pain can be caused by degeneration of the intervertebral disk (diskogenic) or disk height loss leading to segmental instability (degenerative spondylolisthesis). There could also be single- or multisegment facet joint degeneration. All these findings are part of the degenerative cascade as described by Kirkaldy-Willis et al.[2] Thus, a thorough clinical examination would include careful palpation of the lumbar spine, its musculature, and the sacroiliac joints, to look for areas of local tenderness that would help pinpoint pathology. Additional characteristic findings include the presence of an "instability catch" or the patient's experience of a catching pain in the lower back while rising from a forward-leaning posture, which requires supporting their weight by putting their hands on their knees. The patient may also have a "painful catch," in which the raised, straightened leg is unable to move down but suddenly drops due to a sharp pain in the lower back. Both symptoms could point to the presence of spinal instability, likely from a degenerative spondylolisthesis.

Back pain can also result from postural imbalance in both the coronal and sagittal planes. This imbalance is often referred to as the "cone of economy" as discussed by Jean Dubousset.[3] The cone is projected from the feet up, and so the trunk is only within a narrow range. This concept relates to the part of the cone where the body can remain balanced without external support and using minimal effort. The muscular effort required in an upright posture is much greater when the cone is exceeded, and correction should be considered.

Coronal imbalance of the spine can lead to truncal translation and rib-on-pelvis impingement. Sagittal plane deformities include difficulties in standing upright, resulting in muscular fatigue and discomfort from compensating for the global sagittal kyphosis. These global deformities may further stress the sacroiliac and hip joints and lead to buttock and groin pain. Usually the location of the pain is quite accurate in determining the problematic site, but the sacroiliac and hip joints are common sites of misdiagnoses of back pain and should be thoroughly assessed by clinical examination. Shoulder or pelvic asymmetry and shoulder or rib prominence are clues for coronal deformities. Although a forward-leaning posture could be related to muscle fatigue caused by sagittal imbalance, it could also be due to a fixed kyphotic deformity of the spine itself or a result of hip extensor weakness. In addition, during the gait assessment, patients may have worsening kyphotic posture due to muscle decompensation associated with prolonged walking.

Radiological assessment of causes of back pain would require full-length standing posteroanterior and lateral radiographs of the spine, which must include, at a minimum, C7 to the hip joints, but ideally would include C1 to the hip joints, so that balance parameters can be easily measured. Flexion and extension views are useful, and in our experience, standing flexion and prone traction radiographs show the maximum displacement of a spondylolisthesis and its maximum reduction.[4,5] Additional magnetic resonance imaging (MRI) of the lumbar spine is needed to assess neurologic impingement as well as to rule out other causes of back pain. Sometimes, because of the severity of the deformity, a computed tomography (CT) myelogram could be a useful adjunct to identify the exact location of nerve root compression.

Radiological instability is commonly defined by the degree of slip (**Fig. 2.1**), and the change in slip angle (**Fig. 2.2**) and disk height (**Fig. 2.3**). These radiographic features can be found on standing lateral radiographs (degree of slip) and dynamic flexion-extension lateral radiographs (slip angle and disk height). Oblique films can be taken to look for a pars defect. For measurement of the degree of slip, a line is

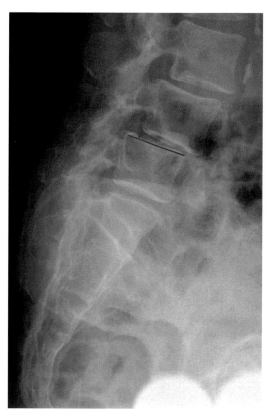

Fig. 2.1 Measurement of the degree of slip. A line is dropped from the posterior border of the cranial vertebrae to the caudal vertebrae. The distance from this point to the posterior border of the caudal vertebrae is divided by the total vertebral body width of the caudal vertebrae. Grade 1 is defined as 0 to 25%, grade 2 is ≥25 to 50%, grade 3 is ≥50 to 75%, and grade 4 is ≥75 to 100%.

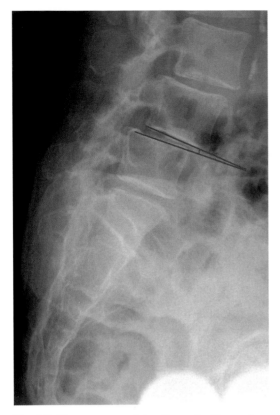

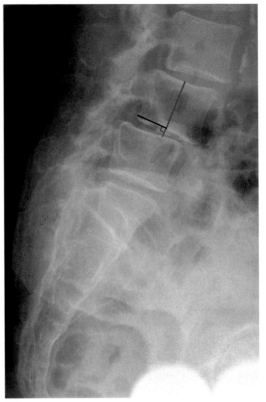

Fig. 2.2 Measurement of the slip angle. The angle is made by the superior end plate of the caudal vertebrae and the inferior end plate of the cranial vertebrae. The slip angle of a L5-S1 spondylolisthesis is measured by a line perpendicular to the posterior aspect of sacrum and a line drawn along the inferior end of the end plate of L5.

Fig. 2.3 Measurement of the disk height. A line is dropped from the midline inferior end plate of the cranial vertebrae to the upper end plate of the caudal vertebrae. The ratio between this distance and the midline vertebral height of the cranial vertebrae is compared on dynamic views.

drawn from the posterior border of the cranial vertebrae to the caudal vertebrae. The distance from this point to the posterior border of the caudal vertebrae is divided by the total vertebral body width of the caudal vertebrae. Grade 1 is defined as 0 to 25%, grade 2 is ≥25 to 50%, grade 3 is ≥50 to 75%, and grade 4 is ≥75 to 100%. Spondyloptosis is defined as more than 100% slip. A slip of greater than 50% is unstable and associated with progression and lumbosacral kyphosis. The slip angle of an L5-S1 spondylolisthesis is measured by a line drawn perpendicular to the posterior aspect of the sacrum and a line drawn along the inferior end of the end plate of L5. In the cranial segments, the slip angle is made by the superior end plate of the

caudal vertebra and the inferior end plate of cranial vertebra. For measuring disk height, a line is drawn from the midline inferior end plate of the cranial vertebra to the upper end plate of the caudal vertebra. A ratio between this distance and the midline vertebral height of the cranial vertebrae is compared on dynamic views. In these cases, fusion surgery is indicated to prevent progression of the instability, correct any segmental deformity, and treat the axial back pain caused by spinal instability.

Full-length standing coronal and sagittal radiographs are used for assessment of the overall coronal and sagittal balance using the center sacral vertical line (**Fig. 2.4**) and C7 plumbline

(**Fig. 2.5**). The bisector of the center sacral vertical line is also useful for finding the proximal neutral vertebra. Sagittal balance is measured by the C7 sagittal plumbline, and lumbar lordosis is usually measured from the upper end plate of T12 to the end plate of S1. Shoulder height, apical vertebral translation of the thoracic and lumbar curves, curve magnitudes, and flexibility should be documented. Common local deformities seen on radiographs include an L2-L3 apex deformity, lateral listhesis or

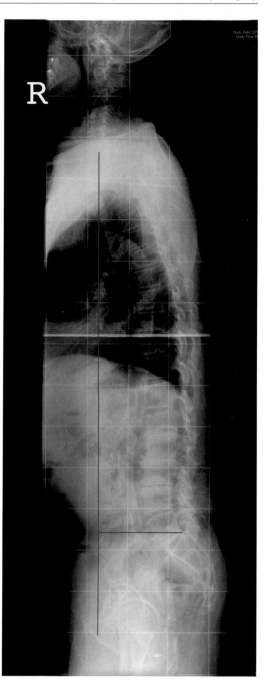

Fig. 2.5 Measurement of sagittal C7 plumb line is done by dropping a vertical perpendicular line to the horizontal from the C7 vertebral body and comparing its horizontal position with the position of the posterosuperior corner of the S1 superior end plate. Sagittal imbalance is normally considered to be > 5 cm deviation from the S1 posterosuperior corner, and in this figure there is a positive sagittal balance.

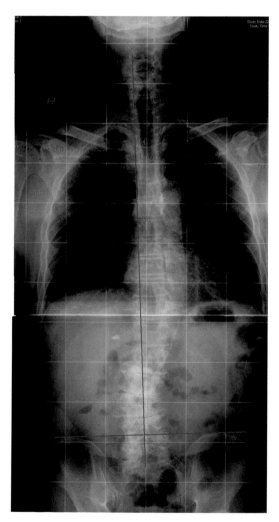

Fig. 2.4 Measurement of central sacral vertical line. Using the top of the iliac crest to control for tilting, a vertical perpendicular line is drawn up from the center of S1. The proximal neutral vertebra can be bisected from this line, and in this figure it would be L2.

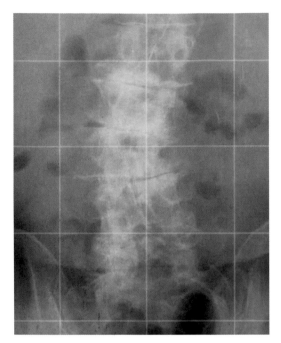

Fig. 2.6 Lateral subluxation is measured by the horizontal distance between the superolateral corner of the caudal vertebra and the inferolateral corner of the cephalad vertebra.

rotatory subluxation (**Fig. 2.6**), lumbar hypolordosis, and short reciprocating curves. Lateral listhesis or rotatory subluxation is measured by the horizontal distance between the superolateral corner of the caudal vertebra and the inferolateral corner of cephalad vertebra. Bending radiographs can differentiate stiff curves from flexible curves, but is more important for deciding on the instrumentation levels during surgery. MRI is useful to assess disk degeneration and spinal stenosis. Deformity correction is required for these symptoms and may require more complex operations such as osteotomies and long fusions.

to vertebral rotatory subluxation, or reduction of the interpedicular distance on the concavity of the curve. These patients usually develop burning or aching pain starting in the buttock that radiates down the appropriately involved dermatome to the lower leg. Clinical identification of the involved dermatome provides a good clue to the likely nerve root affected. This can then be confirmed if there is corresponding weakness in the same myotome. Typically, impingement of the L4 nerve root leads to anterior shin numbness with ankle dorsiflexion weakness (tibialis anterior), an L5 nerve root involves the posterolateral calf and foot dorsum, with extensor hallucis longus weakness, and an S1 nerve root involves the posterior calf and sole, with weakness of the flexor hallucis longus.

Neurogenic claudication commonly presents with insidious onset of buttock, thigh, and calf pain triggered by walking. The usual disability is thus diminished walking tolerance. Vascular claudication is an important differential diagnosis. Patients with vascular claudication may also present with diminished walking tolerance due to calf cramping on exertion or a sensation of tightness that proceeds from distal to proximal. This contrasts to neurogenic claudication where discomfort with numbness proceeds from proximal to distal. Objective sensory examination should pinpoint the specific dermatome or suggest which nerve root is compressed. Motor weakness usually suggests a more long-standing nerve compression. Vascular examination should be performed, including observation for trophic changes in the skin and nails of the lower limbs and diminished distal pulses, which would suggest a vasculogenic cause for the pain.

Radiographic assessment was described above (see Diagnosis of Back Pain).

■ Diagnosis of Leg Pain

The classic presentation of nerve root compression is buttock pain that radiates to the lower extremities and neurogenic claudication. Radicular or leg pain points to spinal or foraminal stenosis caused by facet joint and ligamentum flavum hypertrophy, foraminal narrowing due

■ Factors that May Lead to Curve Progression, Hence the Need for Surgical Treatment

In general, the issue of whether curves progress is debated in the literature, and the rate of progression is highly variable. Curves may progress 1 to 6 degrees per year (average 3 degrees per year).[6,7] Risk factors for progression include a prior history of progression and radiographic risk factors such as asymmetrical disk degeneration, lateral disk wedging, and osteophyte formation.[8-10] Comparing the two sides of a spinal segment, less than 80% of lateral disk wedge and more than 5 mm of lateral osteophyte difference may indicate an unstable segment.[9] Progression has been suggested to occur with Cobb angles greater than 30 degrees, loss of lumbar lordosis, apical rotation larger than Nash-Moe grade 2 (convex pedicle migrates 25% of the vertebral body width and the concave pedicle gradually disappears), lateral listhesis of 6 mm or more, or a prominent or deeply seated L5 disk (in relationship to the intercrestal line).[11-14] The presence of rotatory subluxation, lateral spondylolisthesis, and disk degeneration in the upper lumbar levels also suggests a risk of progressive deformity.[12] Due to spine coupling, rotatory deformity of the spine is related to the development of lateral spondylolisthesis. Thus, apical vertebral rotation may also predict scoliosis progression. Spinal segments proximal to the scoliosis share the load to compensate for spine imbalance. With disk degeneration, this compensatory mechanism fails, and progressive deformity occurs. Fusion surgery is required to prevent curve progression, and the length of fusion is dependent on the presence of coronal or sagittal imbalance.

Management

Management of adult deformities should be tailored to each patient because the symptomatology is different in every case. Treatment is dependent on the experience of the surgeon, the patient's preference, the patient's age and functional status, magnitude of deformity, the rate of progression, and the presence of comorbidities. Sometimes the cause of pain is difficult to differentiate based solely on clinical and radiological examination. In these cases, transforaminal epidural injections, selective nerve root blocks, and facet joint blocks are commonly utilized to identify the pain generator.

Nonoperative management is usually reserved for patients with mild symptoms arising from stenosis, radicular or back pain, curve magnitude of less than 30 degrees, lateral subluxation of less than 2 mm, and reasonable coronal and sagittal balance.[14] Common indications for surgery include axial back pain, symptomatic deformity, neurologic symptoms, and dissatisfaction with appearance. The final decision should be a balance of the magnitude of surgery, the quality of life gain, and the risk of surgical complications. Patients with severe deformity may require major surgery to achieve full correction, and the risk of complications will dramatically increase. Complication rates of up to 80% have been reported in some series.[15,16] Conversely, decompression only or limited fusion may be sufficient to provide reasonable and lasting relief for patients. The following sections discuss the authors' experience in surgical decision making, choosing between decompression only and short or long fusion, and the pitfalls of managing adult deformity.

Critical Factors in Decision Making for Surgery

The goal of surgery for these patients should be to perform the smallest operation possible that would help relieve the symptoms and prevent a recurrence. We find it helps to break down the components of patient complaints in order to make an appropriate decision.

1. Leg pain
   a. Nerve root compression/spinal stenosis—local decompression
   b. Degenerative spondylolisthesis—local decompression ± fusion
2. Back pain
   a. For local degeneration or instability—short fusion
   b. For flexible or correctable sagittal or coronal imbalance—long fusion
   c. For stiff or uncorrectable sagittal or coronal imbalance—long fusion + osteotomies
3. Progressive deformity
   a. Long fusion to prevent progression, seldom would be performed alone in the absence of symptoms above

■ Surgical Decision Making

Decompression Only

Decompression alone is indicated for patients with neurogenic claudication without back pain or a symptomatic or progressive deformity. Decompression is usually in the form of posterior fenestration or laminectomy, although other approaches, including anterior indirect decompression and endoscopic transforaminal approaches, have been described. Each approach has merit and would be dependent on the surgeon's experience. A detailed discussion of their relative merits is beyond the scope of this chapter. As a general principle, in those patients undergoing decompression alone, as much facet joint and as many posterior ligamentous structures as possible should be preserved to reduce the risk of future progression and iatrogenic instability.

One should always be prepared to carry out a local fusion if more extensive bone resection is necessary. This is not uncommon as such individuals often have tight spinal canals, and incidental durotomies are not infrequent. If a wide laminectomy is performed for the repair, a local fusion with pedicle screw fixation may be advisable.

Usual indications for decompression-only surgery include leg pain with minimal or no back pain, Cobb angles of less than 30 degrees, less than 2 mm of lateral subluxation, and normal coronal and sagittal balance indicated by the center sacral vertical line and C7 plumbline.[14] Despite combined back and leg symptoms that may warrant fusion, decompression alone may be indicated for patients with significantly high surgical risk. This may be the best option for an elderly patient with neurogenic claudication, a mild deformity, and poor bone quality. Patients undergoing decompression alone should always be warned of a risk of progression of the deformity that may require a future fusion procedure.

Fusion

Fusion surgery is indicated for the treatment of back pain due to degenerative changes or instability, as well as to prevent progression of the deformity. It may be performed alone or in combination with decompression in patients with radicular symptoms. Short fusion may be useful to stabilize curves with significant apical rotation or when translation or lateral listhesis is greater than 3 mm.[6,12,17,18] However, if there is symptomatic coronal or sagittal imbalance, realignment and long fusion is advisable.

Determination of fusion levels for adult scoliosis is based on the severity of spinal deformity and the global appearance and degenerative changes of the entire spinopelvic axis. There is no universal agreement on the length of fusion and the selection method of the end vertebrae for instrumentation.

Short fusion within the deformity not exceeding the end vertebrae aims to stabilize the spinal segments without correcting the whole deformity. Its major advantage is the lower risk of complications from the anesthesia or the surgery; thus it is indicated in those with back pain but without coronal or sagittal imbalance. Long fusions or fusions extending beyond the end vertebrae is useful for correction of large curvatures with coronal or sagittal imbalance, but this procedure needs to be balanced against increased complication rates.

Typical patients who may be managed with short fusions (**Fig. 2.7**) are those with smaller Cobb angles (less than 30 degrees) and minor rotatory subluxation (lateral subluxations of more than 2 mm).[14] Back and leg pain and segmental instability caused by wide decompressions can all be treated with short fusions.

Long fusions (**Fig. 2.8**), which generally means fusion to L5 or the sacrum, and to T10 or above, yield better surgical correction of the scoliosis and restoration of lumbar lordosis. They are typically indicated for patients whose curves are likely to progress, such as patients with Cobb angles greater than 45 degrees, more than 2 mm of lateral subluxation, and coronal and sagittal imbalance.[14] The aim of the long fusion is to achieve balance in both the coronal and sagittal planes, not absolute Cobb angle correction.[19] Glassman et al[20] demonstrated that positive sagittal balance is the single biggest predictor of clinical symptoms in adult deformity and takes priority over other parameters.

Thus, long fusions should always be considered in patients with global coronal or sagittal imbalance to achieve better functional outcomes.

It should be borne in mind that instrumentation should not end at the level of junctional kyphosis or spondylolisthesis. Any level of severe rotatory subluxation should be included within the fusion block. To balance the spine, the most horizontal vertebra should be the upper instrumented vertebra (UIV).[21] Instrumentation should not end at a level with posterior column deficiency, with listhesis in any direction, at a level of a rotated segment, with junctional kyphosis, at the apex of the deformity in the coronal or sagittal plane, or at a degenerated level.

(*text continues on page 23*)

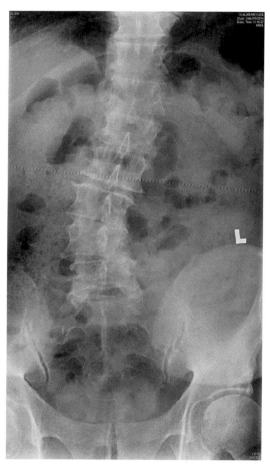

a

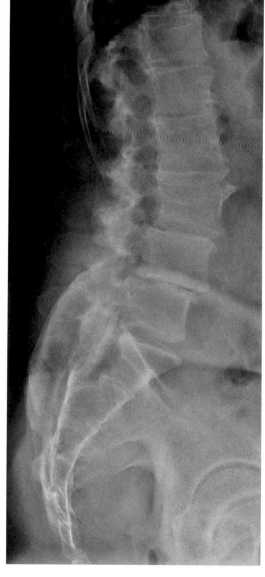

b

Fig. 2.7a–e A 71-year-old man with complaints of axial back pain and bilateral lower limb claudication. **(a)** The patient has degenerative scoliosis from L3 to L5, with a Cobb angle of 25 degrees. **(b)** L3–4 and L4–5 spondylolisthesis and spinal stenosis were noted. (*continued on page 20*)

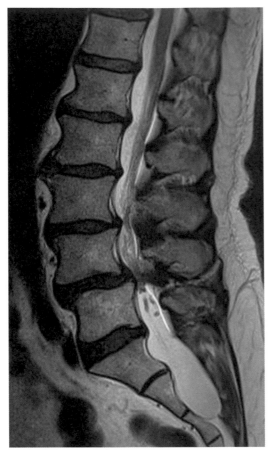

c

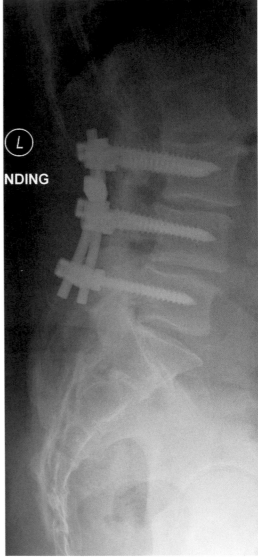

d

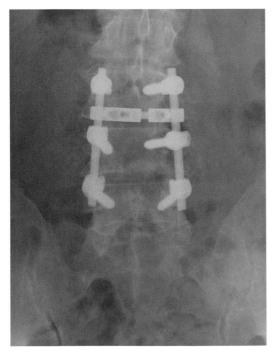

e

Fig. 2.7a–e (*continued*) **(c)** The L5-S1 was well hydrated, and there was no oblique take-off. **(d,e)** Short fusion from L3 to L5 was performed with good correction of the segmental instability.

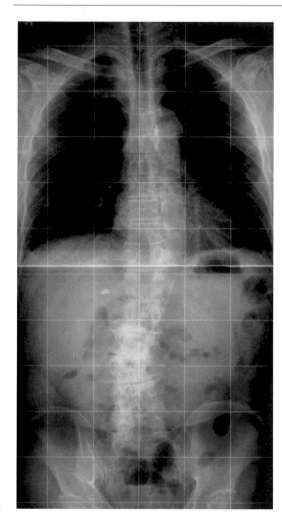

a

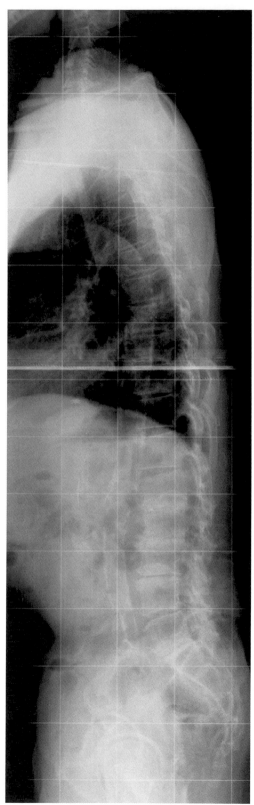

b

Fig. 2.8a–d A 58-year-old man with axial back pain and lumbar hypolordosis. There is **(a)** an oblique L5-S1 with degenerative changes and **(b)** a positive sagittal imbalance. (*continued on page 22*)

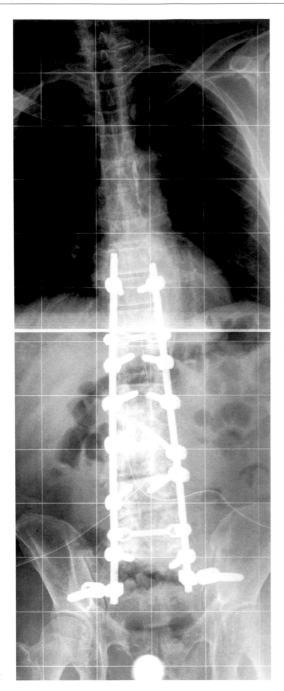

c

d

Fig. 2.8a–d (*continued*) **(c)** The patient was treated with an L3 pedicle subtraction osteotomy and posterior spinal fusion from T10 to the sacrum with S1 and iliac instrumentation. **(d)** Good restoration of sagittal balance is observed postoperatively.

Upper Instrumented Vertebra for Long Fusions

In general, for long fusions, the authors' preference is to end at T10 or above, because instrumentation and fusions ending at T12 to L1 have been shown to have a higher revision rate, likely related to the hypermobile thoracolumbar region as it transitions from an immobile thoracic spine to a mobile lumbar spine. There are also changes in facet orientation from coronal to sagittal and changes in sagittal alignment from kyphosis to lordosis. Extending the UIV to T10 (level with true ribs) or further proximally can provide relative protection to the adjacent segment with the increased stability provided by the rib cage. The rib cage lengthens the transverse dimensions of the spine and gives the thoracic spine greater resistance to bending stresses in multiple planes. T11 or T12 does not have costosternal articulations; hence, these levels lack the biomechanical advantage of the upper levels.

In addition, other factors that could affect long-term survival of that segment need to be taken into consideration. These factors include healthy adjacent spinal segments with no degeneration or instability in any plane, and a UIV adjacent to spinal segments with normal sagittal, coronal, and axial alignment and near-neutral rotation. The UIV should lie within the "stable zone" defined by the center sacral vertical line, before surgery, or could be placed into that zone after surgery.

Currently, there is no consensus study available to recommend T10 instrumentation in all patients to improve long-term results. Disadvantages of the UIV above T10 include increased risk of perioperative complications, and with longer instrumentation across the thoracolumbar spine there is also a greater risk of pseudarthrosis. Thus, the rationale for stopping at T10 may not be applicable in all cases. Important decisions on the extent of instrumentation and fusion should depend on the position of the UIV in relationship to the global spine. An extension to T5 or even higher would depend on the ability of the lumbar surgery to correct the sagittal imbalance. With control of more spinal segments, better sagittal balance may be achieved more easily.

Ultimately, the surgical procedure should be tailored to each patient's needs and based on the goal of achieving a well-balanced, stable, painless, and durable spine with the fewest number of fused segments while reducing the risk of complications associated with large-scale operations.

Lower Instrumented Vertebra for Long Fusions

For the lower instrumented vertebra (LIV), most long fusions will extend to the sacropelvis or stop at L5. In adolescent idiopathic scoliosis, it may be possible to stop at L3 or L4 in a lumbar curve, but because of structural changes and a fixed tilt found at the caudal spinal segments like L4-L5 in adult deformity, stopping at a more cranial segment is generally not advised. Stopping at L5 enables retention of the lumbosacral motion, avoidance of sacroiliac (SI) joint stress, decreased operative time and instrumentation complications, and a lower pseudarthrosis rate. Pelvic fixation can also be avoided. On the other hand, this procedure places a lot of stress at the L5-S1 disk, being the only residual mobile segment, and the patient needs to be warned of future breakdown and the need for surgery to fuse this segment. In general, for many patients, the L5-S1 disk is already degenerated, and in such cases it is probably better to fuse to the sacrum. Preservation of the L5-S1 disk enables some pelvic motion, which may be important for some functional demands of patients, such as riding a bicycle.

Fusion to the sacrum is required for disk degeneration at L5-S1, spondylolisthesis or spinal stenosis at the same segment, as well as oblique take-off at L5-S1 or in fractional curves greater than 15 degrees.[22] Balancing is difficult without fusion down to the sacrum in cases of oblique take-off at L5-S1. In addition, the foramen is smaller on one side, leading to unilateral L5 radiculopathy. It is not uncommon to see patients with foraminal, central, or lateral recess stenosis at L5-S1. If stenosis is present at L5-S1 and more extensive decompression is required, fusing down to the sacrum is inevitable. The obvious disadvantages of fusion to the sacropelvis include increased operative time and more extensive surgical dissection to reach the sacrum. Anterior column support may also be required to reduce the rate of pseudarthrosis. Lost motion at L5-S1 may also alter the patient's gait.

Osteotomies may be required if less than 30% deformity correction can be obtained on bending radiographs. This is not uncommon because adult deformities are usually stiff. To avoid overloading the instrumentation at the metal–bone interface, releases and rebalancing would be required. There are two types of sagittal imbalance in adult deformity. First, the spine is globally balanced but a segmental portion of spine is flat or kyphotic. Second, there is global and segmental imbalance. Coronal imbalance can also be classified into two types with the shoulders and pelvis tilted in opposite directions or with tilting in the same direction. Posterior column osteotomies are the best choice for segmental imbalance of the spine. A prerequisite would be mobile disk spaces to allow extension correction. If the disks are already degenerated and stiff, anterior release is also required. If the bone stock is inadequate, anterior structural grafts can be used to improve fusion rates. For global imbalance, both Smith-Petersen and pedicle subtraction osteotomies can be used. Typically, a Smith-Petersen osteotomy is indicated if the weight-bearing line falls within 3 cm of the sacrum, and a pedicle subtraction osteotomy is reserved for cases with poor bone stock, and it can provide 30 degrees of lordotic correction. In patients with combined coronal and sagittal imbalance, pedicle subtraction osteotomies are a viable option if the shoulders and pelvis are tilted in the same direction, but a vertebral column resection is the better option if the shoulders and pelvis are tilted in opposite directions.

Anterior procedures are required only in rigid deformities that are not passively correctable with posterior instrumentation. They are usually used only in combination with posterior instrumentation, as interbody fusions alone may not be able to correct the overall sagittal alignment.[23] Anterior spinal fusion can further correct lumbar hypokyphosis and imbalance, provide indirect decompression by foraminal distraction, prevent posterior instrumentation failure by load sharing, and decrease the rate of pseudarthrosis, which is especially common in smokers, diabetics, and osteoporotic patients.[14]

Complications

Adult deformity surgery is challenging, and there are many associated complications. Reported complication rates reach 80% for adult deformity, with up to 58% of patients requiring reoperation.[15,16] These degenerative conditions usually occur in the elderly with multiple comorbidities such as pulmonary and cardiac disease, osteoporosis, and nutritional deficiency. These conditions should be properly optimized prior to surgery to decrease perioperative risks. Any of the above comorbidities may affect the timing of surgery as well as the scale of surgical correction.

Deformity correction can indirectly decompress the neural structures by rod derotation, cantilever reduction maneuvers, and particularly by increasing vertebral disk height with anterior interbody fusion. Overdistraction on the concave side may lead to loss of lumbar lordosis. To reduce rigid curves, posterior column osteotomies at multiple levels are likely required to mobilize the spinal segments. Fusions should avoid stopping at a level of rotatory subluxation to prevent aggravating the subluxation.

With limited instrumentation and fusion, degeneration may be accelerated in the remaining curve as a result of adjacent segment disease. Stopping the fusion within the deformity may provoke these adjacent segment problems. Stopping the fusion at the thoracolumbar junction also leads to adjacent segment disease cranial to the segment of fusion. Fusion to T10 or above may avoid this. However, some consider adjacent segment degeneration unpreventable in fusion surgery as it could be due to the natural age-related progression of a degenerative process coupled with the postsurgical effect of spinal stiffening created by fusion or instrumentation procedures.[24,25]

Proximal adjacent segment degeneration is detected by progressive narrowing of disk height, progressive decrease in lordosis or increase in kyphosis, osteophyte formation, sclerosis of an adjacent end plate, or translation in the coronal or sagittal planes. Proximal junctional problems such as adjacent segment degeneration, compression fracture, or screw failure in the UIV occurs more frequently with fusions ending at T11 to L2 as compared with those at T10 or above.[26]

For the LIV, depending on fusion to L5 or to the sacrum, different complications may occur, including L5-S1 disk degeneration, loss of curve and balance correction, iliac screw implant problems, and pseudarthrosis. If the fusion is stopped at L5 where there is fixed sagittal imbalance and disk degeneration at L5-S1, the rate of disk degeneration will further increase, leading to loss of sagittal profile correction and L5-S1 spondylolisthesis.[22] In osteoporotic bone, fusion to L5 has a high risk of fixation failure, as the L5 pedicles are mostly cancellous and there are trajectory problems in obtaining a medial angle for placing the pedicle screws. Failure of L5 screws with loosening leads to kyphosis or hypolordosis of the L4-L5 segment. L4-L5 kyphosis may be tolerated in a short fusion, but with longer fusions the degree of sagittal imbalance becomes an issue.

Fusions to the sacrum should be reserved for L5-S1 spondylolisthesis, stenosis, oblique takeoff, moderate or severe L5-S1 degeneration, and prior laminectomy. Problems with long fusions to the sacrum include higher complication rates due to a large-scale operation, risk of sacroiliac joint degeneration, altered gait mechanics and increased pseudarthrosis. Instrumentation complications for these long fusions include breakage and back-out or loosening of screws. To avoid this, S1 screws should be bicortical through the promontory anteriorly. S1 screws should also be directed medially to avoid penetrating the L5 nerve root. Bone grafting anterior to L5-S1 and iliac screws may further protect the S1 fixation. To improve the L5-S1 fixation, distal hooks, iliac screws, and interbody cages for anterior column support are also options. Hooks are an alternative fixation especially in osteoporotic bone but may cause stenotic problems at L5-S1.

Iliac screws entail the risk of pullout[27] and are usually more prominent. Screws should be buried if possible, but, in thin patients, removal may be required and should be done around 2 years after fixation. Technically, iliac screws are more difficult to insert with previous posterior iliac bone harvesting. There is also a higher pseudarthrosis rate at L5-S1, but this may be salvaged by revision surgery with anterior reconstruction and iliac fixation as well as using bone morphogenetic protein to improve fusion rates. The lowest pseudarthrosis rate of L5-S1 fusions is associated with complete sacropelvic fixation and surgery in patients younger than 55 years of age.[28]

■ Chapter Summary

In adult deformity, there is difficulty in matching a patient's symptoms and concerns with the surgical plan. Clinicians must weigh potential gains and risks, and all surgical decisions should be individually tailored to the patient. Comorbidities should be addressed prior to surgery to avoid perioperative complications. Usually, the surgical options include decompression alone, decompression with limited arthrodesis, and deformity correction with long fusion (**Table 2.1**). Decompression surgery is reserved for patients with leg pain but minimal or no back pain, scoliosis Cobb angles less than 30 degrees, less than 2 mm of subluxation, no thoracic hyperkyphosis, and acceptable coronal and sagittal balance, or if they have a poor premorbid state. For short fusions, patients should have scoliosis Cobb angles less than 30 degrees, segmental instability (more than 2 mm of lateral subluxation), back and leg pain, no significant imbalance issues, and, if destabilizing, decompression is required for adequate relief of spinal stenosis and nerve root compression. Long fusions are reserved for scoliosis Cobb angles greater than 45 degrees, more than 2 mm of subluxation, and coronal and sagittal imbalance. To avoid complications related to instrumentation,

Table 2.1 Decompression Surgery Only Versus Short Fusion Versus Long Fusion

Symptom or Condition	Decompression Only	Short Fusion	Long Fusion
Pain	Radicular pain, minimal or no back pain	Back and leg pain	Back and leg pain
Scoliosis	Cobb angle < 30 degrees	Cobb angle < 30 degrees	Cobb angle > 30 degrees
Subluxation	< 2 mm	< 2 mm	> 2 mm
Overall balance	Acceptable coronal and sagittal balance	Acceptable coronal and sagittal balance	Global coronal and sagittal imbalance
Stability	Stable motion segment	Segmental instability, > 50% pars/facet excision for decompression	Segmental and regional kyphosis
Operated levels	Stenotic levels only	Rotatory subluxation segments within fusion block, segmental instability caused by wide decompression	UIV: T10 LIV: L5 if no degeneration, spondylolisthesis, stenosis or oblique take-off at L5-S1
Limitations	Cannot address global balance, progressive deformity, segmental instability with wide decompression	Higher surgical risk, cannot address global balance, adjacent level disease	Highest surgical risk, compromised fixation with osteoporosis, high risk of pseudarthrosis, iliac screw prominence

Abbreviations: UIV, upper instrumented vertebra; LIV, lower instrumented vertebra.

fusion should not end at a level with junctional kyphosis or spondylolisthesis, posterior column deficiency, a rotated segment, a level at the apex of the deformity, or a degenerated level. Levels of rotatory subluxation must be included within the fusion block. For balance, the most horizontal vertebra should be the UIV. Extension of the fusion to T10 provides the increased stability offered by the rib cage. The LIV at L5 is only feasible with a normal L5-S1 disk, and no spondylolisthesis or spinal stenosis or oblique take-off at L5-S1. Fusions to the sacrum should be avoided if possible to avoid iliac screw implant problems, pseudarthrosis, sacroiliac joint problems, and gait disturbances, but is usually mandatory for long-standing sagittal and or coronal imbalances.

Pearls

◆ All surgical decisions for degenerative scoliosis should be individually tailored to the patient.
◆ Decompression surgery is reserved for patients with leg pain, minimal or no back pain, scoliosis

Cobb angles less than 30 degrees, less than 2 mm of subluxation, no thoracic hyperkyphosis, acceptable coronal and sagittal balance, or those with poor premorbid state.
◆ Short fusions are for scoliosis Cobb angles less than 30 degrees, segmental instability, back and leg pain, and no significant imbalance issues.
◆ Long fusions are for scoliosis Cobb angles greater than 45 degrees, more than 2 mm of subluxation, and coronal and sagittal imbalance.
◆ Extension of the fusion to T10 provides increased stability offered by the rib cage.
◆ The most horizontal vertebra should be the UIV.

Pitfalls

◆ Fusion should not end at a level with junctional kyphosis or spondylolisthesis, posterior column deficiency, a rotated segment, at the apex of the deformity, or a degenerated level.
◆ Avoid the LIV ending at L5 with an abnormal L5-S1 disk, spondylolisthesis, spinal stenosis, or oblique take-off at L5-S1.
◆ Fusions to the sacrum should be avoided if possible due to the increased risk of iliac screw implant problems, pseudarthrosis, sacroiliac joint problems, and gait disturbances.

References
Five Must-Read References

1. Schwab F, Dubey A, Gamez L, et al. Adult scoliosis: prevalence, SF-36, and nutritional parameters in an elderly volunteer population. Spine 2005;30:1082–1085

2. Kirkaldy-Willis WH, Wedge JH, Yong-Hing K, Reilly J. Pathology and pathogenesis of lumbar spondylosis and stenosis. Spine 1978;3:319–328

3. Dubousset J. Three-dimensional analysis of the scoliotic deformity. In: Weinsteid S, ed. The Pediatric Spine: Principles and Practice. New York: Raven Press; 1994

4. Luk KD, Cheung KMC. Lumbar spinal instability. Hong Kong Journal of Orthopaedic Surgery 1998;2

5. Luk KD, Chow DH, Holmes A. Vertical instability in spondylolisthesis: a traction radiographic assessment technique and the principle of management. Spine 2003;28:819–827

6. Bradford DS, Tay BK, Hu SS. Adult scoliosis: surgical indications, operative management, complications, and outcomes. Spine 1999;24:2617–2629

7. Grubb SA, Lipscomb HJ, Coonrad RW. Degenerative adult onset scoliosis. Spine 1988;13:241–245

8. Benner B, Ehni G. Degenerative lumbar scoliosis. Spine 1979;4:548–552

9. Jimbo S, Kobayashi T, Aono K, Atsuta Y, Matsuno T. Epidemiology of degenerative lumbar scoliosis: a community-based cohort study. Spine 2012;37:1763–1770

10. Kobayashi T, Atsuta Y, Takemitsu M, Matsuno T, Takeda N. A prospective study of de novo scoliosis in a community based cohort. Spine 2006;31:178–182

11. Grubb SA, Lipscomb HJ. Diagnostic findings in painful adult scoliosis. Spine 1992;17:518–527

12. Pritchett JW, Bortel DT. Degenerative symptomatic lumbar scoliosis. Spine 1993;18:700–703

13. Robin GC, Span Y, Steinberg R, Makin M, Menczel J. Scoliosis in the elderly: a follow-up study. Spine 1982;7:355–359

14. Silva FE, Lenke LG. Adult degenerative scoliosis: evaluation and management. Neurosurg Focus 2010;28:E1

15. Carreon LY, Puno RM, Dimar JR II, Glassman SD, Johnson JR. Perioperative complications of posterior lumbar decompression and arthrodesis in older adults. J Bone Joint Surg Am 2003;85-A:2089–2092

16. Edwards CC II, Bridwell KH, Patel A, Rinella AS, Berra A, Lenke LG. Long adult deformity fusions to L5 and the sacrum. A matched cohort analysis. Spine 2004;29:1996–2005

17. Sapkas G, Efstathiou P, Badekas AT, Antoniadis A, Kyratzoulis J, Meleteas E. Radiological parameters associated with the evolution of degenerative scoliosis. Bull Hosp Jt Dis 1996;55:40–45

18. Tribus CB. Degenerative lumbar scoliosis: evaluation and management. J Am Acad Orthop Surg 2003;11:174–183

19. Simmons ED. Surgical treatment of patients with lumbar spinal stenosis with associated scoliosis. Clin Orthop Relat Res 2001;384:45–53

20. Glassman SD, Berven S, Bridwell K, Horton W, Dimar JR. Correlation of radiographic parameters and clinical symptoms in adult scoliosis. Spine 2005;30:682–688

21. Simmons ED Jr, Simmons EH. Spinal stenosis with scoliosis. Spine 1992;17(6, Suppl):S117–S120

22. Bridwell KH. Selection of instrumentation and fusion levels for scoliosis: where to start and where to stop. Invited submission from the Joint Section Meeting on Disorders of the Spine and Peripheral Nerves, March 2004. J Neurosurg Spine 2004;1:1–8

23. Cho KJ, Suk SI, Park SR, et al. Short fusion versus long fusion for degenerative lumbar scoliosis. Eur Spine J 2008;17:650–656

24. Ghiselli G, Wang JC, Bhatia NN, Hsu WK, Dawson EG. Adjacent segment degeneration in the lumbar spine. J Bone Joint Surg Am 2004;86-A:1497–1503

25. Kumar MN, Baklanov A, Chopin D. Correlation between sagittal plane changes and adjacent segment degeneration following lumbar spine fusion. Eur Spine J 2001;10:314–319

26. Shufflebarger H, Suk SI, Mardjetko S. Debate: determining the upper instrumented vertebra in the management of adult degenerative scoliosis: stopping at T10 versus L1. Spine 2006;31(19, Suppl):S185–S194

27. Weistroffer JK, Perra JH, Lonstein JE, et al. Complications in long fusions to the sacrum for adult scoliosis: minimum five-year analysis of fifty patients. Spine 2008;33:1478–1483

28. Kim YJ, Bridwell KH, Lenke LG, Rhim S, Cheh G. Pseudarthrosis in long adult spinal deformity instrumentation and fusion to the sacrum: prevalence and risk factor analysis of 144 cases. Spine 2006;31:2329–2336

3

The Use of Osteotomies for Rigid Spinal Deformities

Stephen J. Lewis and Simon A. Harris

■ Introduction

The use of spinal osteotomies in severe spinal deformities has enabled corrections that were not considered possible in the past. With advanced posterior-based techniques, excellent corrections are achieved through a single approach, shortening the duration of surgery and reducing the need for multiple position changes during surgery. Although the majority of corrections can be performed from the posterior direction, selective deformities may require combined anterior procedures.

With the improvement in surgical techniques and neuromonitoring modalities, obtaining corrections of severe spinal deformities is now both possible and reasonably safe.[1] Thorough knowledge of advanced anatomy, careful preoperative planning, and specialized instrumentation and implants provide the necessary tools for successful surgery. This chapter reviews the various osteotomies, the indications for their use, as well as the methods of maximizing corrections and minimizing both short- and long-term complications.

■ Planning the Deformity Correction

Although deciding whether or not to operate is the first main decision to be made, planning the finer details of the procedure will help ensure a smoother flow of the surgery. The main planning should be done preoperatively, and an algorithm for key decisions should be established preoperatively and discussed with the patient and family. For example, if the patient does not wish to assume the increased risk associated with achieving a more complete deformity correction, it is important to discuss what can be achieved with lesser releases. Conversely, if correction is a key component of the patient's expectations and the surgical team can reliably achieve these goals safely, a three-column osteotomy can be performed if lesser osteotomies are unsuccessful.

Determining the Flexibility of the Deformity

Using the least risky procedure to obtain a correction is key to the safe outcome of deformity surgery. If a similar correction can be obtained through multiple posterior column releases, a three-column osteotomy may not be necessary. Determining the flexibility of the curve can often be difficult, and intraoperative adjustments may be required in cases where the curve is more stiff or less stiff than expected.

Helpful clues to curve flexibility include the presence of wide disk spaces, disk spaces that open and close on bending films, and curve magnitudes that decrease when the patient is in the prone position or with traction views. If computed tomography (CT) imaging demonstrates anterior fusions, either congenital or from previous surgery, these fusions will not correct with posterior releases, and three-column osteotomies will be required. In contrast, good corrections can be achieved with posterior column releases through previous posterior fusion masses that have not undergone previous anterior fusions. Proper preoperative workup with long-cassette anteroposterior (AP) and lateral side benders, CT scan, and magnetic resonance imaging (MRI) should be done preoperatively, so that the best possible preoperative plan can be made. Newer technologies with three-dimensional (3D) printers can provide surgeons with preoperative models of the spine, to even better prepare for the ultimate procedure.

Exposure

Excellent exposure is an essential component of the procedure. Severe deformities can make this more challenging; however, taking the time to obtain the necessary exposure will greatly facilitate implant insertion, and generally improve the flow of the procedure. It is important to identify the spine levels, areas with previous decompressions, fusion masses, and previous implants. In cases of revisions, knowledge of previous spinal instrumentation will ensure that the required instruments are available to facilitate implant removal.

Spinal Cord Blood Flow

The blood flow to the spinal cord enters the dura through vessels that travel with the exiting nerve root. Although nerve roots are commonly sacrificed in thoracic-level osteotomies, taking a nerve root at the level of the artery of Adamkiewicz could lead to significant detriment to the spinal cord circulation.[2] This artery has variable anatomy, but is present between T8 and L1 on the left side in the majority of people. When considering osteotomies around the thoracolumbar junction, protecting and saving the nerve roots may preserve key sources of blood flow.

For thoracolumbar three-column osteotomies, preoperative angiography can be performed to determine the exact location of the artery of Adamkiewicz. The artery runs a characteristic intradural "hairpin" loop on imaging[3] (**Fig. 3.1**). The location of the artery may influence the choice of level of the osteotomy, and the surgeon may choose a level other than the apex if the artery is present at the apex. Injuring this vessel, especially in the presence of

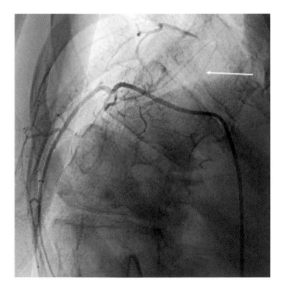
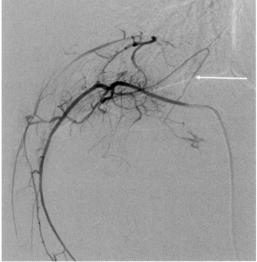

b

Fig. 3.1a,b Spot image **(a)** and inverse **(b)** shots of angiography of the left T11 segmental artery showing the characteristic intradural hairpin loop *(white arrow)*, representing the artery of Adamkiewicz. In this patient, the vessel enters the dura through the left T11 foramen and forms the loop that extends up to T10. With the vessel arising two levels proximal to the apex, a vertebral column resection was performed at L1 without incident.

hypotension, can lead to a loss of intraoperative motor evoked potential (MEP) monitoring that is often delayed from the time of injury. With spinal cord infarction as one of the main risks of spinal cord level osteotomies, knowledge of and attention to this artery may help prevent this devastating complication, especially in patients with previous anterior procedures, where segmental vessels may have been ligated.

Fixation

Achieving adequate and stable fixation is essential to obtaining and maintaining deformity correction. Although the pedicle screw is the main anchor in the majority of constructs, alternatives such as hooks, laminar screws, fusion mass screws or hooks, wires, and bands should be considered when pedicle screw fixation is not possible.[4] Obtaining adequate proximal anchors is generally the key determinant of successful constructs in thoracic osteotomies. Osteotomies should not be attempted unless solid proximal and distal fixation is established. Careful planning from the preoperative images will help to identify and select the appropriate anchor for each level.

During osteotomy closure, various methods can be utilized to protect the main implants. Temporary devices or implants can be used to close the osteotomies, such as central rod constructs, sparing the main screws.[5] The use of periapical reduction screws, tubes, or other extenders on the screws, linking of multiple anchors to the rod before cantilevering the reduction, and the use of a three- or four-rod technique with connectors can facilitate reduction of the osteotomy and correction of the deformities while protecting the main anchors.

Determining the Desired Correction

The imaging should be carefully studied to identify the deformity and determine the type and magnitude of the desired correction. Careful understanding of the normal sagittal alignment, the pelvic parameters, and the magnitude

of the deformity will help to identify which osteotomies would be required to gain the desired correction.[6,7]

For fixed kyphotic deformities, correction will be achieved through anterior lengthening, posterior shortening, or a combination of both. For coronal deformities, correction will be achieved through concave lengthening, convex shortening, or a combination of both. For fixed lordosis, correction can be achieved through anterior shortening, posterior lengthening, or a combination of both. For multiplanar deformities, it is important to identify the primary deformity or deformities, and tailor an osteotomy or combination of maneuvers to achieve the desired correction. For example, for a fixed kyphotic scoliosis, a combination of posterior shortening and convex shortening could be the primary mode of correction. If a vertebral column resection (VCR) were to be performed, a larger anterior cage placed on the concavity could maximize correction. For fixed hyperlordosis, a formal anterior release or resection could be combined with posterior column releases to achieve the desired correction.[8]

The magnitude of the deformity must be considered. Rough estimates of potential correction through a single osteotomy include 10 degrees of sagittal or coronal plane correction through a single posterior column release, 30 to 35 degrees of sagittal and 10 to 15 degrees of coronal plane through a single pedicle subtraction osteotomy (PSO), and 30 to 50 degrees of correction through a VCR in the coronal or sagittal plane.[9,10] For a VCR, more correction will be achieved through a deformity without a previous fusion compared with one that is previously fused, as correction will be achieved only through the osteotomy site and not through the adjacent segments in cases of previous fusion masses. Properly estimating the desired correction relative to the deformity will help plan the number and types of osteotomies required to achieve the desired correction.[11]

Deciding the Level of the Osteotomy

For posterior column releases (Smith Petersen, Ponte), multiple periapical osteotomies will help achieve a gradual, multilevel correction for deformities with mobile anterior columns. For three-column osteotomies (PSO, PSO variants, VCR), the preferred vertebra would be at the apex of the deformity, not tilted in the coronal or sagittal planes, and would be appropriate for proximal and distal fixation. Other considerations include the location of the artery of Adamkiewicz and the presence of pseudarthrosis in cases of revisions, in which cases it would preferable be include the nonfused levels in the osteotomy.

Planning an Osteotomy

Putting all the information together will help to determine the best option for deformity correction. A representative case is a 66-year-old woman with ankylosing spondylitis (**Fig. 3.2**). Preoperative imaging with long-cassette radiographs and CT demonstrated the autofusion of her spine. Her chief complaints are sagittal imbalance and difficulty with forward gaze. Her pelvic incidence measures 55 degrees, the lumbar lordosis 10 degrees, with a sacral slope of 5 degrees and a pelvic tilt of 50 degrees. With the desired lumbar lordosis being 10 degrees less than the pelvic incidence, and the desired pelvic tilt being less than 25 degrees, she would require ~ 35 degrees of lumbar lordosis. This can best be achieved through a single lumbar PSO.

As for her thoracic spine, she has significant complaints related to her gaze. Her thoracic kyphosis from T5 to T12 measures 25 degrees, which is within the normal range. Her T2-T5,

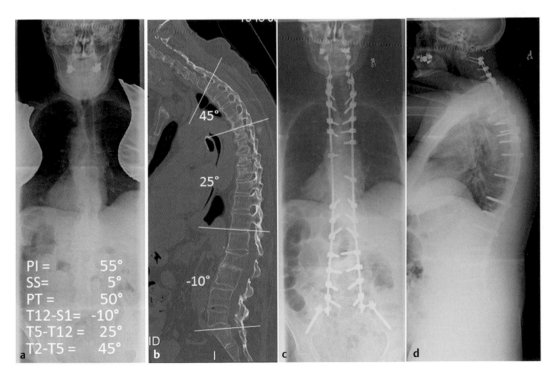

Fig. 3.2a–d Representative case of a 66-year-old woman with ankylosing spondylitis as demonstrated on the preoperative standing posteroanterior radiograph **(a)** and the sagittal CT reconstruction **(b)**. Abnormal sagittal alignment is characterized by a low sacral slope (SS), high pelvic tilt (PT) and insufficient lumbar lordosis (LL, T12-S1) for the given pelvic incidence (PI). To maintain a balanced relationship of the PI and LL, an L2 pedicle subtraction osteotomy (PSO) was performed. Forward gaze was improved with a T3 PSO to correct the proximal thoracic kyphotic deformity. Stabilization of this correction was achieved with a C2 to pelvis construct as demonstrated on the standing postoperative long-cassette posteroanterior **(c)** and lateral **(d)** radiographs.

however, measures 45 degrees, which is greater than the 10 to 15 degrees expected for this region. A single PSO in this region would provide the necessary correction to improve her gaze.

This patient underwent a T3 and an L2 PSOs with a C2-to-pelvis stabilization through a single-stage procedure, addressing both of her deformities and providing her with the necessary sagittal balance.

Single Procedure or Staged

Although it may be preferable to complete the surgery in one stage, certain factors may necessitate performing the procedure in two or more stages. These factors include excessive bleeding, long duration of the surgery, medical comorbidities, and difficulties with neuromonitoring. Recognizing these difficulties preoperatively may help to electively plan performing these surgeries over two separate days. The benefits of staging include minimizing operative team fatigue, postponing the bleeding portion of the procedure to the second day, and the possibility of obtaining proper imaging to check the position of the instrumentation prior to the second stage. The timing between stages is controversial. Some advocate a short time of 1 to 2 days, whereas others recommend 1 to 2 weeks to allow patients to achieve their normal nutritional status before proceeding. Logistical issues of operative time and surgical team availability, as well as patient and family issues, also need to be considered in the decision.

The Surgical Team

Having a strong, cohesive surgical team with open communication is essential to the success of these complex reconstructions. Ideally, the team should include an experienced spine surgeon and anesthesiologist, skilled surgical assistants, a nursing team familiar with the instrumentation and procedure, an experienced neuromonitoring and radiology technologist, and a blood conservation team. Open communication is important, and such issues as blood pressure parameters, blood conservation strategies, neuromonitoring changes, and informa-

tion about the surgical field and the stage of the procedure should be reviewed frequently throughout the case.[12]

Obtaining Fusion Across the Osteotomy

Obtaining a solid fusion across the osteotomy is important in preventing early implant failure at the level of the osteotomy. Although multiple rods can increase the rigidity of the constructs, having stable anterior and posterior columns with bridged structural bone across all defects is key to obtaining fusion. Anterior grafts are not sufficient to overcome large posterior column defects. Resected ribs can be preserved in the procedure and used to bridge posterior column defects following osteotomy closure.[13] Techniques of fashioning the rib and the host bed, wiring ribs in place, or using mini-screws from the craniofacial internal fixation sets to secure the ribs will help re-create the structural continuity of the posterior column.

■ Osteotomy Options

Spinal osteotomies can be divided into six main types[14] (**Fig. 3.3**):

Posterior column:
1. Partial facet
2. Complete facet

Partial body:
3. Pedicle subtraction osteotomy (PSO)
4. Transdiskal pedicle subtraction osteotomy

Complete body:
5. Vertebral column resection (VCR)

Multiple vertebrae:
6. Multiple vertebral column resection

In this classification, the approach modifier was added. If the procedure was performed from posteriorly, the osteotomy would have a "P" after the number. If a combined anterior and posterior surgery was performed, an "A/P" would be added after the number. For example, if a PSO was performed from posteriorly, it would be considered a type 3P osteotomy. A VCR performed through a combined anterior

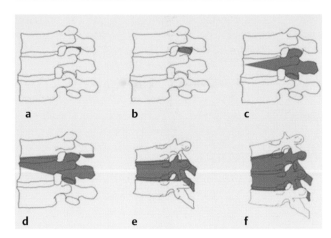

Fig. 3.3a–f Schematic of the comprehensive anatomic spinal osteotomy classification proposed by Schwab et al. In this classification, Type 1 (**a**) is a partial facet resection, type 2 (**b**) is a complete facet resection, type 3 (**c**) is a pedicle subtraction osteotomy, type 4 (**d**) is a transdiskal pedicle subtraction osteotomy, type 5 (**e**) is a vertebral column resection, and type 6 (**f**) is a multi-level vertebrectomy. (From Schwab F, Blondel B, Chay E, et al. The comprehensive anatomical spinal osteotomy classification. Neurosurgery 2014;74:112–120, discussion 120. Reprinted with permission.)

and posterior approach would be considered a type 5 A/P.

Types 1 and 2: Posterior Column Osteotomies

Release of the facet joints and the posterior ligamentous structures, including the ligamentum flavum, provides significant mobility to the posterior column. For any correction to occur, the anterior column has to be mobile. With the combination of a mobile anterior column and a released posterior column, significant correction can be achieved in both the coronal and sagittal planes (**Fig. 3.4**). For kyphosis correction, this osteotomy provides a combination of posterior shortening and anterior lengthening.

Type 1 osteotomies involve resection of the inferior facets. This can provide some mobility in the posterior column. Type 2 osteotomies involve removal of the superior facet and ligamentous structures. Resection of the superior facet is the key to the release. This can be achieved without resecting the inferior facets,

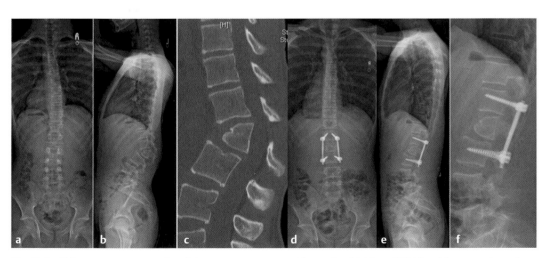

Fig. 3.4a–f Long cassette standing (**a**) posteroanterior, (**b**) lateral, and (**c**) sagittal computed tomography (CT) reconstruction of a 17-year-old boy with an L2 congenital kyphosis. Note the global compensation of the deformity through thoracic and lumbar hyperlordosis. Posterior column osteotomies were performed at L1-L2 and L2-L3, with correction of the deformity and stabilization from (**d**) L1 to L3, allowing for (**e**) the spontaneous normalization of the thoracic kyphosis and a decrease in (**f**) the compensatory lumbar hyperlordosis.

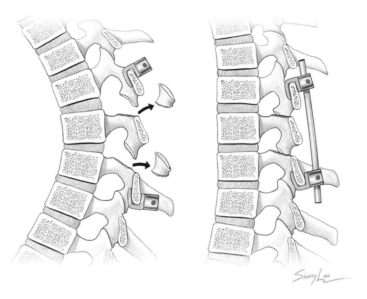

a
b

Fig. 3.5a,b (a) Schematic of a posterior column osteotomy with resection of the superior facets. **(b)** Osteotomy closure is achieved with a temporary central hook-rod construct reducing the inferior facet to the proximal surface of the pedicle. Note the flexible anterior column allowing anterior lengthening with osteotomy closure. (From Lewis SJ, Goldstein S, Bodrogi A, et al. Comparison of pedicle subtraction and Smith-Petersen osteotomies in correcting thoracic kyphosis when closed with a central hook-rod construct. Spine 2014;39:1217–1224. Reprinted with permission.)

especially when significant distraction of the facets occurs, as is the case with large kyphotic deformities. Preservation of the inferior facet during the osteotomy can help to maintain posterior-column bone stock, aiding in the posterior fusion. Use of a hook-based temporary central rod to facilitate osteotomy closure following the posterior column release produced ~ 10 degrees of correction per osteotomy level in the thoracic spine (**Fig. 3.5**).

Type 3: Pedicle Subtraction Osteotomy

The PSO is a posterior-based closing-wedge osteotomy. It is ideally suited for kyphosis correction and can reliably produce 25 to 35 degrees of lordosis even in the presence of a solidly fused anterior column[15] (**Fig. 3.6**). Performing the PSO asymmetrically can enable concomitant coronal plane correction. A PSO can be performed in both the thoracic and lumbar spines. In cases of pelvic incidence (PI) and lumbar lordosis (LL) mismatch with an as-

sociated abnormally high PI, a sacral PSO can be performed to decrease the PI and normalize the PI–LL relationship.[16]

The main complications associated with PSOs are bleeding, potential nerve root injury or entrapment, and pseudarthrosis. The technique is discussed below. Careful attention to detail can help minimize the potential morbidity that can be seen with these cases.

Technique

Multiple variations of the technique have been described, but the principles of the procedure are common to all of them.

Decompression

Following exposure and implant insertion, the pedicle is isolated from all of its bony attachments: laterally, the transverse process; distally, the pars; and proximally, the superior facet. A complete laminectomy of the involved level is performed as well as of some or all of

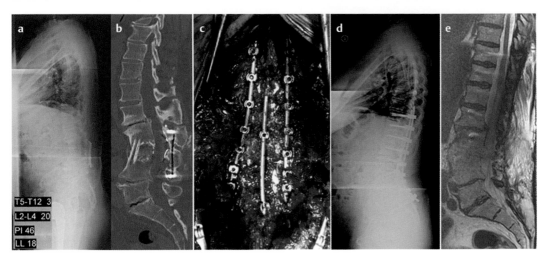

Fig. 3.6a–e Long cassette standing **(a)** lateral and **(b)** sagittal CT reconstruction of a 67-year-old man who underwent a previous anterior and posterior L2-L4 fusion for an L3 burst fracture. Intraoperative views with **(c)** the temporary central rod in place and postoperative long cassette **(d)** lateral and **(e)** sagittal T2 magnetic resonance imaging (MRI) demonstrating restored sagittal alignment following an L3 PSO and T10 to pelvis construct.

the adjacent levels to ensure adequate space for the dural sac centrally upon closure. Complete resection of the pedicle is required to create a single foramen for two nerve roots—the nerve root of the osteotomy level as well as the nerve root of the level proximal. The complete posterior elements of the vertebra of the osteotomy level should be resected. A triangular posterior-based wedge of bone is then removed from the body, leaving a small amount of anterior bone of the vertebral body. The anterior column acts as a hinge during closure.

For thoracic-level osteotomies, the transverse processes are removed to reveal the medial rib. The rib is dissected free from all its soft tissue attachments, taking care to avoid entering the pleural space. The rib is then cut 5 to 6 cm lateral from the vertebra. Subperiosteal dissection is done to free up the medial rib, which is then detached from the lateral aspect of the vertebral body. Dissection along the lateral pedicle and body is then performed to free the mediastinum from the ventral vertebral body. Spoon retractors can then be placed around the anterior vertebra to further protect the mediastinal structures. Retracting the spinal cord should be avoided during the decompression to minimize iatrogenic injury.

Minimizing Bleeding During the Osteotomy

The epidural veins run a predictable course; identifying, coagulating, and cutting them can minimize blood loss during the procedure. The veins run through the epidural fat and should be coagulated while separating the fat from the dura. A second series of veins run along the medial aspect of the pedicle, distally along the course of the exiting nerve root and proximally over the pedicle and deep to the superior facet. When reaching around ventrally, care should be made to avoid the segmental vessels running along the midportion of the lateral vertebral body. As well, failure to separate the plane of the mediastinum from the ventral body can lead to significant mediastinal venous bleeding during dissection lateral to the vertebral body. It is imperative to stay along the lateral aspect of the vertebra when dissecting anteriorly.

Osteotomy Closure

Closure of the osteotomy is performed after ensuring adequate resection of the posterior wall of the vertebral body and after complete resection of the pedicles has been performed. If difficulty is encountered closing the osteotomy, the surgeon should consider resecting more bone anteriorly for adequate decompression. Inadequate bone resection is the main reason osteotomies do not close.

To judge the reduction of the posterior column, the inferior facet of the level proximal to the osteotomy can be preserved and reduced to the superior facet of the level distal to the osteotomy. This will ensure a stable posterior column with structural bone continuity and prevent overshortening during closure. Closure can be achieved through the use of a hook-based central rod (**Fig. 3.7**), through compression of the periapical anchors with temporary short rods, or with three- or four-rod constructs using side-to-side rod connectors. If posterior column continuity cannot be achieved through osteotomy closure, structural bone graft (from adjacent ribs or large spinous processes) can be used to fill the posterior defects.

Type 4: Transdiskal Variant

Modifying the proximal resection of the PSO to extend across the disk space provides for a greater resection and enables bone-on-bone contact through the anterior column. This variation is particularly useful in cases of diskitis with kyphotic collapse (**Fig. 3.8**) and posttraumatic kyphosis.[17]

PSO with Previous Anterior Implants

Anterior implants at the level of the planned osteotomy present a challenge when performing posterior-based procedures. The implants can be removed either through a formal anterior approach or through an anterior reach-around procedure from a posterior approach[18] (**Fig. 3.9**). Posteriorly the transverse processes are removed, and dissection is performed along the lateral aspect of the pedicle. The anterior implants are identified. Taking care to preserve the exiting nerve root, a metal cutting bur can be used to cut the anterior rod proximal and distal to the anterior screw. Some of the lateral body is then removed to identify the neck of the screw, which is then cut with the bur. The segment of the anterior screw with the attached rod is removed. The osteotomy is then

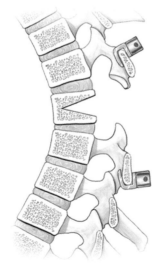

a

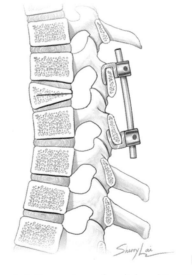

b

Fig. 3.7a,b Schematic of **(a)** a pedicle subtraction osteotomy closed with **(b)** a central rod. Note the reduction of the inferior facet of the proximal level to the superior facet of the distal level, re-creating a new facet joint and continuity of the posterior column. (From Lewis SJ, Goldstein S, Bodrogi A, et al. Comparison of pedicle subtraction and Smith-Petersen osteotomies in correcting thoracic kyphosis when closed with a central hook-rod construct. Spine 2014;39:1217–1224. Reprinted with permission.)

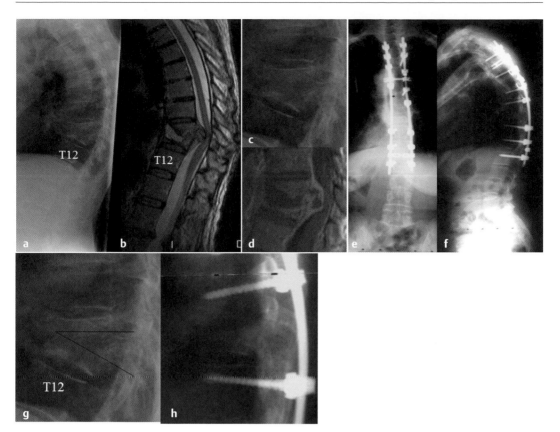

Fig. 3.8a–h Long cassette **(a)** lateral and **(b)** sagittal T2-weighted MRI of a 73-year-old woman with known tuberculosis unresponsive to medical treatment. Note the destruction and kyphotic collapse of the T10-T11 disk space and **(c)** adjacent vertebral bodies with an associated epidural abscess noted on **(d)** gadolinium-enhanced T1-weighted MRI. Long cassette **(e)** posteroanterior and **(f)** lateral views demonstrate a T4 to L2 posterior reconstruction. **(g)** A transdiskal pedicle subtraction osteotomy was performed by resecting the posterior elements and pedicles of T11, the proximal vertebral body of T11, the T10-T11 disk, and the distal vertebral body and end plate of T10. **(h)** A new vertebral body was creating by reducing the proximal body of T10 to the distal vertebral body of T11. Note the inferior facet of T10 was reduced to the superior facet of T12 to maintain the integrity of the posterior column.

performed in the usual fashion and the remaining shaft of the screw is removed with the vertebral body resection (**Fig. 3.10**).

Type 5: Vertebral Column Resection

For large multiplanar deformities, resection of a complete vertebral body can provide the mobility in the spine to achieve the needed correction.[19] Severe kyphotic deformities, like those seen following tuberculosis, often require more extensive resections involving multiple vertebrae to achieve the needed correction. Common indications for VCR include severe kyphoscoliosis, congenital deformities (**Fig. 3.11**), and rigid deformities secondary to previous surgery.[20]

The procedure is performed in a similar fashion to a PSO. Although the PSO is often performed for primarily sagittal plane deformities, the VCR can accommodate multiplanar deformities. These deformities often have major rotational and translational components, causing

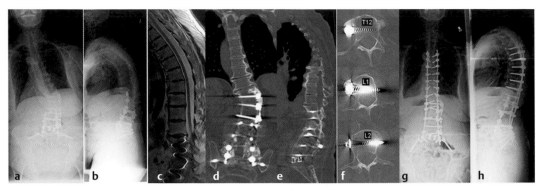

Fig. 3.9a–h Long cassette **(a)** posteroanterior and **(b)** lateral view, sagittal T2 MRI **(c)**, and CT coronal **(d)**, sagittal **(e)**, and representative axials **(f)** of a 69-year-old woman with coronal and sagittal malalignment following a previous anterior T12 to L5 fusion and circumferential extension to the sacrum and pelvis. Thoracic kyphosis (T5-T12) measures 45 degrees, lumbar lordosis (T12-S1) measures 7 degrees, the pelvic incidence measures 51 degrees, the sacral slope measures 5 degrees, and the sagittal vertical axis measures 12 cm. **(g,h)** The patient underwent an offset L2 pedicle subtraction osteotomy through a posterior approach and proximal extension to T4, as demonstrated in the standing postoperative long-casette posteroanterior **(g)** and lateral **(h)** ragiographs. The L2 anterior screw was removed from the same posterior approach.

significant challenges to the exposure, the dissection, and the decompression, especially on the concave side (**Fig. 3.12a,b**). Care must be taken when dissecting around the vertebral body on the concavity, to ensure that the dissection does not enter the mediastinum. Similarly, with the severe rotation, the spinal cord will be shifted against the concavity (**Fig. 3.12c,d**), making it vulnerable to injury with removal of the concave pedicle. These challenges are not as difficult when performing a PSO for sagittal plane deformities.

The steps for a VCR are similar to those for a PSO: exposure, followed by insertion of implants, removal of the transverse processes, removal of the medial ribs and rib heads, exposure

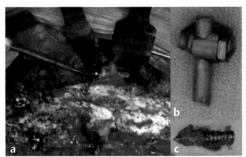
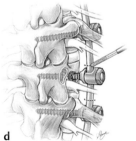
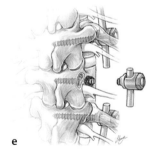

Fig. 3.10a–e **(a)** Intraoperative view of the lateral and anterior dissection performed to identify the previously placed anterior instrumentation through a posterior exposure. Note the preservation of the exiting nerve root. A metal-cutting high-speed drill is used to cut the anterior rod proximal and distal to the screw. After removal of some of the lateral vertebral body, a further cut is made along the neck of the screw. **(b)** The screw head with the attached rod is removed. **(c)** The shaft of the screw is extracted when completing the osteotomy. **(d,e)** A schematic demonstrates the removal of the anterior implant. (From Lewis SJ, David K, Singer S, et al. A technique of anterior screw removal through a posterior costotransversectomy approach for posterior-based osteotomies. Spine 2010;35: E471–E474. Reprinted with permission.)

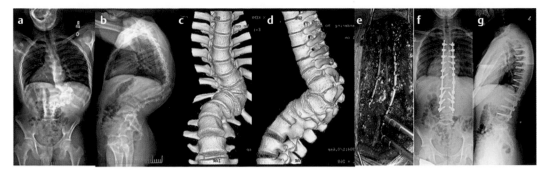

Fig. 3.11a–g **(a)** Anteroposterior and **(b)** lateral long cassette radiographs of a 19-year-old man with congenital kyphoscoliosis. **(c,d)** Three-dimensional reconstructions demonstrates a T11 hemivertebra at the apex of the deformity. The patient underwent **(e)** posterior resection of T11 and T12 and **(f,g)** posterior reconstruction from T5 to L4. A portion of the resected vertebra was used as an anterior strut between T10 and L1 to maintain the integrity of the anterior column. Closure of the osteotomy was performed with proximal to distal convex rod placement with the temporary concave rod, with loosened set screws in place to prevent translation.

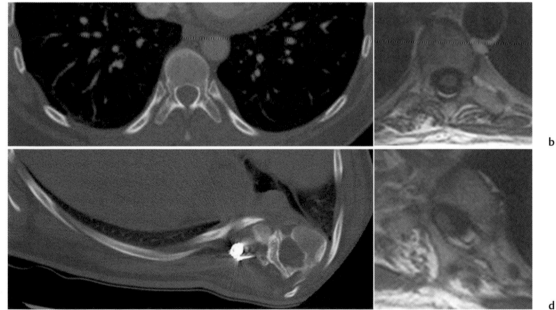

Fig. 3.12a–d Axial **(a)** CT and **(b)** MRI of a non-rotated thoracic spine with kyphosis. Note the position of the rib heads and the central position of the spinal cord. **(c)** Comparative CT of a patient with a severe scoliosis. Note the marked rotation of the vertebra, the convex lateral vertebral body abutting the posterior aspect of the convex rib, the very ventral position of the concave rib, and the posterior position of the convex rib head. **(d)** Axial MRI shows the spinal cord shifted against the concave rib.

of the ventral vertebral body, posterior decompression, removal of the concave pedicle, temporary concave rod, convex removal of the pedicle, and release of the proximal and distal disks. The vertebral body can be removed piecemeal or en bloc. For piecemeal removal, a shell of ventral vertebral body cortex can be left behind to protect the mediastinal structures and serve as a barrier for the anterior strut graft or cage. For en-bloc resection, circumferential release of the disks needs to be performed to permit adequate release and removal. Release of the concave side of the disk is the most difficult. Often the adjacent medial ribs on the concavity need to be removed to provide sufficient access for the release. The tap for the pedicle screws can be used as a joystick from the convexity to facilitate the complete removal of the vertebral body. The use of proper retractors to protect the mediastinal structures during anterior body resection is paramount.

When performing VCR with marked rotation, it is easiest to enter the canal through the convex foramen to start the decompression. The complete posterior elements of the level to be resected should be removed, along with the laminae of the adjacent levels. This will provide good visualization of the spinal cord upon osteotomy closure. The concave pedicle is carefully removed and a temporary rod is then placed on the concavity. The majority of the remaining dissection and vertebrectomy can be performed from the convexity without the temporary rod being in the way.

A structural anterior support graft, either a part of the resected vertebra or a cage, is inserted anteriorly to guide the reduction and prevent overshortening. A laminar spreader can be used to distract ventrally from the concave side to facilitate the graft/cage insertion. Closure of the VCR should be done with a convex rod. The temporary concave rod is left in place, with the set screws loosened, preventing translation without hindering osteotomy closure. Reduction is often easiest from proximal to distal. Single- and dual-rod reduction techniques have been described. Reducing a proximal and distal convex rod to a central connector has also been described. Being familiar with multiple techniques and the equipment available will enable the surgeon to tailor the method to the given situation.

Type 6: Multilevel Vertebral Column Resection

Severe kyphotic angular deformities, often secondary to remote infections, are amenable to posterior-based vertebral resections. A single level is often insufficient. Multiple levels of the remnants of the deformed vertebrae are resected (**Fig. 3.13**). Following resection, ventral distraction aids in lengthening the anterior column for placement of an anterior cage/strut. Posterior shortening through the rod will complete the correction.

■ Osteotomies for Fixed Lordosis

The correction of fixed hyperlordosis requires a combination of anterior shortening and posterior lengthening. This is most reliably accomplished through a formal anterior release followed by a posterior correction (**Fig. 3.14**). Similar to severe kyphosis, where the vertebral column is displaced posteriorly, in fixed hyperlordosis the spine is displaced ventrally. This ventral displacement favors an anterior approach, with the spine being superficial to the anterior abdominal wall. In cases of thoracic hyperlordosis, severe narrowing of the mediastinum occurs, with bronchial compression occurring in the more severe cases. Even in cases with respiratory issues, these patients paradoxically benefit from formal anterior approaches to decrease the lordosis and help increase the kyphosis, thereby increasing the anteroposterior diameter of the mediastinum, relieving the bronchial compression.

Anterior shortening can be accomplished with multiple-level diskectomies for global hyperlordosis or through resection of disk and bone for more focal deformities (**Figs. 3.15** and **3.16**). A posterior-column release and instrumentation is then performed. Contouring the posterior rod in the appropriate sagittal plane will then reduce the lordotic deformity. Formal

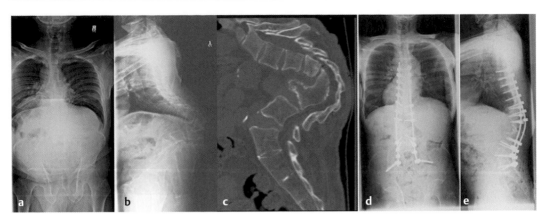

Fig. 3.13a–e **(a)** Anteroposterior and **(b)** lateral views of a 59-year-old man with severe kyphosis secondary to remote infection. **(c)** CT sagittal view shows four vertebrae autofused ventrally with a severe focal kyphosis, and hyperlordosis of the distal lumbar and thoracic spines. **(d,e)** Long cassette radiographs demonstrating correction following multilevel vertebrectomy, placement of an anterior cage, and posterior T6 to pelvis instrumentation.

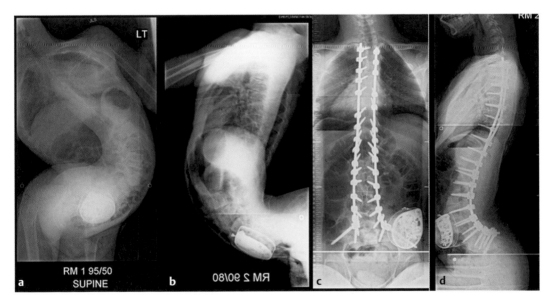

Fig. 3.14a–d Supine **(a)** anteroposterior and **(b)** lateral long cassette radiographs of a 17-year-old boy with severe neuromuscular lordoscoliosis with previous Baclofen pump insertion. **(c,d)** Following L1 to S1 anterior diskectomies, intraoperative traction and a posterior T2 to pelvis instrumentation and fusion was performed.

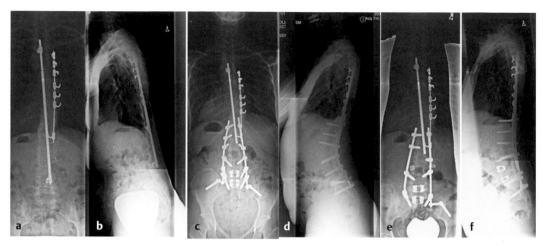

Fig. 3.15a–f (a) Anteroposterior and **(b)** lateral long cassette radiographs of a 47-year-old woman with a remote Harrington rod instrumentation and fusion for adolescent idiopathic scoliosis. She presented with distal degeneration and sagittal malalignment. **(c,d)** An L3 pedicle subtraction osteotomy and anterior lumbar interbody fusions at L4–5 and L5-S1 were performed, resulting in fixed lumbar hyperlordosis. Because of the patient's severe unhappiness with her sagittal alignment, an anterior L2–3 diskectomy and resection of the proximal portion of the L3 vertebral body followed by a L2–3 posterior column release were performed. The posterior fusion mass release was gently distracted and held open with mesh cages, while an appropriately contoured rod was inserted from distal to proximal to reduce the osteotomy. **(e,f)** This resulted in a more balanced sagittal plane. (From Lewis SJ, Gray R, David K, Kopka M, Magana S. Technique of Reverse Smith Petersen osteotomy (RSPO) in a patient with fixed lumbar hyperlordosis and negative sagittal imbalance. Spine 2010;35: E721–E725. Reprinted with permission.)

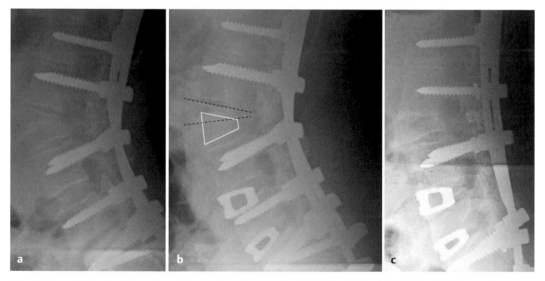

Fig. 3.16a–c Lateral radiographs of the patient in **Fig. 3.15** demonstrating **(a)** the L3 pedicle subtraction osteotomy and **(b)** the planned resection for the reverse Smith–Petersen osteotomy. **(c)** Close-up lateral view of the lumbar spine following closure of the combined anterior/posterior osteotomy. (From Lewis SJ, Gray R, David K, Kopka M, Magana S. Technique of Reverse Smith Petersen osteotomy (RSPO) in a patient with fixed lumbar hyperlordosis and negative sagittal imbalance. Spine 2010;35:E721–E725. Reprinted with permission.)

posterior distraction after the circumferential release may cause unwanted distraction of the entire spine instead of just the posterior column, making the reduction to an under-contoured rod the preferred method.

■ Chapter Summary

The approach to severe spinal deformities has significantly changed with the improved techniques, imaging, and instrumentation that are available. An improved outcome will be achieved with careful preoperative planning, a deep understanding of the deformities, and the knowledge and ability to perform the various correction techniques. Creating an environment with experienced and skilled surgical and perioperative teams will help to predict and manage the complexities associated with the successful treatment of these challenging cases.

Pearls

◆ Obtaining appropriate preoperative imaging studies can help to better understand the complexities of the deformity and the patient's anatomy, and to plan for potential difficulties in the procedure.

◆ Careful preoperative clinical and radiographic evaluation will help to assess the flexibility of the deformity, to determine the fixation options, and to decide on the location, number, and type of osteotomies required to achieve the desired correction.

◆ Accurate intraoperative spinal cord monitoring, including motor evoked potentials, is essential to the safe completion of these procedures. Understanding the timing and magnitude of neuromonitoring changes will direct key intraoperative decisions.

◆ Although pedicle screw instrumentation is the primary method of curve control, alternative fixation methods such as fusion mass screws or laminar hooks are important backup strategies, especially in revision surgery or dysplastic anatomy.

Pitfalls

◆ The artery of Adamkiewicz has a variable anatomy from T8 to L1, most commonly on the left side. When considering osteotomies around the thoracolumbar junction, protecting and saving the nerve roots may preserve key sources of blood flow.

◆ Careful and controlled reduction of three-column osteotomies is essential to prevent cord translation and subsequent injury. Complete visualization of the cord and harmonious collaboration with the surgical team, electrophysiological monitoring team, and nursing staff is essential for spinal cord safety.

References
Five Must-Read References

1. Dorward IG, Lenke LG. Osteotomies in the posterior-only treatment of complex adult spinal deformity: a comparative review. Neurosurg Focus 2010;28:E4

2. Dommisse GF. The blood supply of the spinal cord. A critical vascular zone in spinal surgery. J Bone Joint Surg Br 1974;56:225–235

3. Boll DT, Bulow H, Blackham KA, Aschoff AJ, Schmitz BL. MDCT angiography of the spinal vasculature and the artery of Adamkiewicz. AJR Am J Roentgenol 2006;187:1054–1060

4. Lewis SJ, Arun R, Bodrogi A, et al. The use of fusion mass screws in revision spinal deformity surgery. Eur Spine J 2014;23(Suppl 2):181–186

5. Lewis SJ, Goldstein S, Bodrogi A, et al. Comparison of pedicle subtraction and Smith-Petersen osteotomies in correcting thoracic kyphosis when closed with a central hook-rod construct. Spine 2014;39:1217–1224

6. Schwab F, Patel A, Ungar B, Farcy J-P, Lafage V. Adult spinal deformity-postoperative standing imbalance: how much can you tolerate? An overview of key parameters in assessing alignment and planning corrective surgery. Spine 2010;35:2224–2231

7. Rose PS, Bridwell KH, Lenke LG, et al. Role of pelvic incidence, thoracic kyphosis, and patient factors on sagittal plane correction following pedicle subtraction osteotomy. Spine 2009;34:785–791

8. Lewis SJ, Gray R, David K, Kopka M, Magana S. Technique of Reverse Smith Petersen osteotomy (RSPO) in a patient with fixed lumbar hyperlordosis and negative sagittal imbalance. Spine 2010;35:E721–E725

9. Cho K-J, Bridwell KH, Lenke LG, Berra A, Baldus C. Comparison of Smith-Petersen versus pedicle subtraction osteotomy for the correction of fixed sagittal imbalance. Spine 2005;30:2030–2037, discussion 2038

10. Dorward IG, Lenke LG, Stoker GE, Cho W, Koester LA, Sides BA. Radiographic and clinical outcomes of posterior column osteotomies in spinal deformity correction. Spine 2014;39:870–880

11. Bridwell KH. Decision making regarding Smith-Petersen vs. pedicle subtraction osteotomy vs. vertebral column resection for spinal deformity. Spine 2006;31(19, Suppl):S171–S178

12. Jarvis JG, Strantzas S, Lipkus M, et al. Responding to neuromonitoring changes in 3-column posterior spinal osteotomies for rigid pediatric spinal deformities. Spine 2013;38:E493–E503

13. Lewis SJ, Kulkarni AG, Rampersaud YR, et al. Posterior column reconstruction with autologous rib graft after en bloc tumor excision. Spine 2012;37:346–350

14. Schwab F, Blondel B, Chay E, et al. The comprehensive anatomical spinal osteotomy classification. Neurosurgery 2014;74:112–120, discussion 120

15. Lafage V, Schwab F, Vira S, et al. Does vertebral level of pedicle subtraction osteotomy correlate with degree of spinopelvic parameter correction? J Neurosurg Spine 2011;14:184–191

16. Lafage V, Bharucha NJ, Schwab F, et al. Multicenter validation of a formula predicting postoperative spinopelvic alignment. J Neurosurg Spine 2012;16:15–21

17. Halpern EM, Bacon SA, Kitagawa T, Lewis SJ. Posterior transdiscal three-column shortening in the surgical treatment of vertebral discitis/osteomyelitis with collapse. Spine 2010;35:1316–1322

18. Lewis SJ, David K, Singer S, et al. A technique of anterior screw removal through a posterior costotransversectomy approach for posterior-based osteotomies. Spine 2010;35:E471–E474

19. Hamzaoglu A, Alanay A, Ozturk C, Sarier M, Karadereler S, Ganiyusufoglu K. Posterior vertebral column resection in severe spinal deformities: a total of 102 cases. Spine 2011;36:E340–E344

20. Lenke LG, O'Leary PT, Bridwell KH, Sides BA, Koester LA, Blanke KM. Posterior vertebral column resection for severe pediatric deformity: minimum two-year follow-up of thirty-five consecutive patients. Spine 2009;34:2213–2221

4

Indications and Techniques for Sacral-Pelvic Fixation in Adult Spinal Deformity

Kristen E. Jones, Robert A. Morgan, and David W. Polly, Jr.

▪ Introduction

Fusion attempts across L5/S1 in adult spinal deformity are plagued by a high rate of pseudarthrosis and implant breakage/failure due to the unique anatomic and biomechanical characteristics of the lumbosacral junction.[1,2] In a single-institution review of adult deformity patients with constructs greater than four levels, constructs ending at S1 had a significantly higher rate of pseudarthrosis compared with constructs ending at L5 or more cephalad levels.[1] Other pseudarthrosis risk factors were age older than 55 years, more than 12 levels included in the construct, and T10-L2 kyphosis of greater than 20 degrees. The addition of sacral-pelvic fixation increases the strength and stability of constructs spanning the lumbosacral junction and is a formidable tool in the spinal deformity surgeon's armamentarium for correcting spinal imbalance.

▪ Anatomic and Biomechanical Considerations

As a transition zone from the mobile lumbar spine to the stiff pelvis, the lumbosacral junction experiences significant forces challenging arthrodesis attempts across the segment. Despite bearing axial loads of more than double body weight, the osseous anatomy of the sacrum provides relatively little strength for fixation.[3] The sacrum consists of a thin rim of cortical bone surrounding a cancellous core, with large pedicle diameter precluding the engagement of both medial and lateral cortical walls via pedicle screw instrumentation.

The lumbosacral junction is a biomechanically distinct location that is subjected to the highest level of translational shear force and the most limited range of motion within the spine, with the L5/S1 disk bearing the largest summation of load vectors.[2,4–6] These unique stresses, combined with the relatively small amount of sacral cortical bone available for fixation, result in increased pseudarthrosis and implant breakage/failure in long instrumentation constructs ending at S1.[2,7]

McCord et al[6] introduced the concept of the lumbosacral pivot point at the junction of the L5-S1 disk and the middle osteoligamentous column to describe the considerable flexion moments and cantilever forces acting at the lumbosacral junction. Extending fixation anterior to this pivot point increases construct strength. Screw insertion into the ilium provides the longest fixation length anterior to this pivot point, and was found to be the only instrumentation type at the lumbosacral junction that significantly increased the maximum flexion moment at failure. Compared with the weak cancellous composition of the sacrum, the posterior ilium offers abundant cortical bone for anchoring instrumentation and enables increased screw length and diameter, making sacral-pelvic fixation a useful technique for increasing construct strength.

■ Indications for Sacral-Pelvic Fixation

The rigid fixation provided by sacral-pelvic instrumentation is a useful adjunct to treating a wide array of pathological entities. Sacral-pelvic fixation is indicated for lumbosacral arthrodesis extending cephalad to the L2 vertebra, augmentation for poor quality or osteoporotic bone, sacrectomy for tumor or infection, unstable sacral fractures, correction of flat-back syndrome via lumbar osteotomy, correction of pelvic obliquity, and high-grade spondylolisthesis.[8] The addition of iliac fixation in these conditions significantly reduces the stress placed on S1 instrumentation and increases construct strength.

As with all spinal surgery, selection of the appropriate approach for each individual patient and meticulous attention to surgical technique is the key to successful treatment. Although sacral-pelvic fixation is not required for many patients undergoing lumbosacral arthrodesis, the force vectors required for the creation and maintenance of proper sagittal alignment relative to the patient's individual bone quality must be considered.

■ Sacral-Pelvic Instrumentation Selection and Techniques

Sacral Fixation

Screws at S1 can be placed through the pedicles in a medially convergent manner with bicortical end-plate or tricortical purchase, or through the ala in a divergent manner (**Fig. 4.1a**). Sublaminar hooks and wires and S2 pedicle screws can be used to supplement S1 pedicle/alar screws but should not be relied on for anchoring a long construct.

S1 Pedicle Screws

The sizable medially convergent sacral pedicles accommodate large screw length and diameter while simultaneously preventing "filling" the pedicle to achieve bicortical purchase of the medial and lateral pedicle wall with a single screw. The largely cancellous sacral pedicles provide relatively little pullout strength in unicortical fixation, and unicortical pedicle screws should be avoided.[3] Bicortical fixation anchored into the anterior sacral cortex provides increased pullout strength compared with unicortical S1 pedicle screws; however, additional trajectories can be employed to further enhance pullout strength. Luk et al[9] compared bicortical S1 pedicle screw insertion torque and pullout strength to that of S1 pedicle screws advanced through the S1 superior end plate. S1 pedicle screws traversing the end plate had significantly higher insertional torque and pullout strength compared with bicortical S1 screws.

Tricortical fixation, defined as a screw trajectory toward the medial sacral promontory, captures purchase in the dorsal, anterior, and superior end-plate cortex (**Fig. 4.1b**). Lehman et al[10] found that this tricortical trajectory doubles the insertional torque compared with bicortical S1 pedicle screws parallel to the S1 end plate. Tricortical S1 screw strength has not been directly compared with trans–end-plate screw strength; both provide enhanced strength compared with typical bicortical purchase parallel to the S1 end plate. Triangulation of the pedicle screw trajectory increases pullout strength compared with straight-ahead trajectory and should be universally employed.

Sacral Alar Screws

Alar screw insertion utilizes a lateral trajectory into low-density cancellous sacral bone. Bicortical alar fixation is technically possible but fraught with risk of injuring the L5 nerve roots

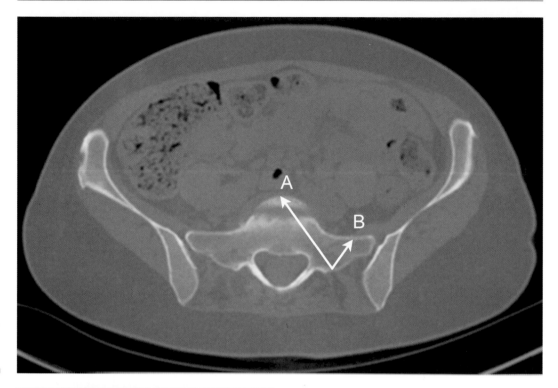

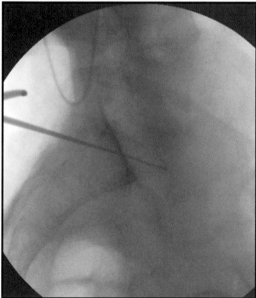

Fig. 4.1a,b Sacral screw trajectories. **(a)** Trajectories for S1 pedicle (A) and alar (B) screw placement. **(b)** Intraoperative view demonstrating probe insertion in tricortical S1 screw trajectory. Tricortical purchase utilizing dense sacral promontory cortical bone should be employed to maximize screw pullout strength.

or common iliac vessels draped anteriorly across the ala.[3] Thus, alar screws are utilized mainly as unicortical supplements to bicortical/tricortical S1 pedicle screw constructs. A Chopin or Colorado plate or a Tacoma block can be utilized to connect S1 and alar screws. Disadvantages of this technique include constrained screw starting point and potential impairment of the ideal trajectory.

Sacral Sublaminar Wires and Hooks

Although sublaminar wires and hooks lack sufficient biomechanical strength to serve as anchors to long constructs, they can be used as supplements for short-segment fusions.[3,11] Hooks are optimally placed in the dorsal sacral neuroforamina where improved cortical purchase can be achieved. The Harrington instrumentation system initially employed sacral hooks as anchors to long constructs, but the rate of pseudarthrosis and hook dislodgment at L5/S1 was unacceptably high. Sacral sublaminar wires and hooks should not be used as anchors to long constructs.

S2 Screws

S2 pedicle screw strength is typically limited by a short pedicle length and a location dorsal to the lumbosacral pivot point described by McCord et al[6] and Kebaish.[11] S2 pedicle screws and S2 screws directed laterally into the ala can be used as adjunct support to short-segment fusions but lack the biomechanical strength to anchor long constructs.[12]

Jackson Intrasacral Rod Technique

Jackson intrasacral rods are inserted vertically through the ala from S1 to the level of S2 and then can be connected to a construct including S1 pedicle screws. Insertion is technically difficult and can be precluded by alar anatomic variations. This technique has been shown to be biomechanically inferior to a lumbosacral pedicle screws–iliac screw construct and is mentioned for historical context only.[5]

Transsacral Fixation

Kellogg Speed first described transvertebral strut grafting at L5/S1 from an anterior approach for patients with high-grade spondylolisthesis. The Speed technique involves driving a fibular strut graft through the L5 vertebral body and into the sacrum via anterior exposure, and is a useful technique in lieu of interbody cage placement, which has an increased risk of anterior subsidence for patients with high-grade spondylolisthesis.[13]

Due to the risk of the anterior exposure to the lumbosacral junction, including injury to the great vessels during mobilization or sympathetic plexus dysfunction causing retrograde ejaculation in males, H.H. Bohlman popularized the posterior approach for transvertebral fibular strut grafting at L5-S1 for patients with high-grade spondylolisthesis. Anterior fixation through L5/S1 can also be performed via a paracoccygeal approach in a minimally invasive fashion utilizing synthetic implants. As with all constructs, the addition of posterior column support increases stability.

Iliac Fixation

Anchoring a construct with iliac fixation creates a longer lever arm to resist cantilever forces across the lumbosacral junction via extension anterior to the lumbosacral pivot point, increasing biomechanical strength of sacral-pelvic constructs.[6] Incorporation of the ilium into a construct offloads stress from sacral screws and decreases the rate of sacral instrumentation failure and pseudarthrosis across the lumbosacral junction.[4,14]

Transiliac Fixation

Harrington Threaded Sacral Rod

Developed for pelvic fixation in adjunct with Harrington distraction rods, this device is mentioned for historical purposes. Two separate posterior iliac incisions are used to insert the threaded rod through the posterior iliac wings with compression applied. Pseudarthrosis rates have been reported above 40%m and the distraction forces of Harrington rods can result in sagittal plane imbalance.[2,8]

Kostuik Transiliac Bar

Inserted from the midline, the Kostuik transiliac bar is placed 1 to 2 cm anterior to the posterior superior iliac spine and then attached via custom connectors to S1 pedicle or alar screws. The bar is smooth and has a contoured shape that accommodates the midline sacral dorsal prominence, and has been reported to have a high fusion rate of up to 97%.[8]

Iliac Fixation

Luque L-fixation

The first to develop segmental instrumentation, Luque extended lumbosacral constructs to the pelvis using L-shaped rods whose ends were inserted into the posterior ilium at the posterior superior iliac spine. This circumvented the distraction problem associated with the Harrington technique and improved fusion rates, but pistoning occurring between the rods decreased the stability of the Luque L-fixation in torsion and flexion.[2,8]

Galveston Technique

Ben L. Allen and Ron L. Ferguson developed the Galveston technique in the 1980s. Smooth rods inserted from the posterior superior iliac spine into the ilium were connected to segmental lumbosacral instrumentation. Rod contouring required significant expertise. To obviate the need for this, rods with pre-bent sagittal contour and bilateral iliac fixation were created in a single piece.[3] This construct still required substantial rod management skills. Because the smooth rods had inferior pullout strength compared with threaded screws, iliac screws quickly became a more popular method of fixation.

Iliac Screws

Iliac fixation with single or stacked unilateral or bilateral screws is performed with fully or partially threaded screws. The pullout strength and rotational stability is superior to non-threaded rod techniques. The starting point for screw insertion is at the level of the posterior superior iliac spine with a trajectory targeting either the supra-acetabular notch or the anterior superior iliac spine (**Fig. 4.2**). The screw trajectory is planned via visualization of the "iliac teardrop" on either fluoroscopy or computed tomography (CT) image guidance. The iliac teardrop is a region above the acetabulum bordering the medial iliac wall, the lateral iliac wall, and the zenith of the sciatic notch. The screw achieves greatest purchase in the lateral margin of the teardrop, directed through the cortical bone just above the sciatic notch. Santos et al[15] analyzed various screw lengths and diameters and found a significant increase in insertional torque for iliac screws of length ≥ 80 mm and diameter ≥ 9.5 mm. No difference in insertional torque existed between the supra-acetabular notch and the anteroinferior iliac spine directed trajectory. Given the risk of acetabular joint violation with the supra-acetabular trajectory, the authors concluded that optimal iliac screws are inserted in the anteroinferior iliac spine trajectory with length ≥ 80 mm and diameter ≥ 9.5 mm.

Iliac screws can be used in combination with sacral screws to provide increased construct strength and are biomechanically superior to other pelvic fixation options. Comparing the Galveston technique to iliac screws in a series of 20 neuromuscular scoliosis patients, iliac screws enabled better correction of pelvic obliquity and decreased implant breakage.[16]

In a biomechanical comparison between the modified Galveston technique with iliac fixation but no S1 fixation versus S1 pedicle screws plus iliac screws, or S1 and S2 screws without iliac fixation, Tis et al[17] found that constructs with iliac screws conferred significant strength via decreased range of motion in multidirectional flexibility testing and increased load to failure.

Bridwell's group[4] performed a laboratory investigation comparing multidirectional flexibility and flexural load to failure among the following construct types: lumbosacral pedicle

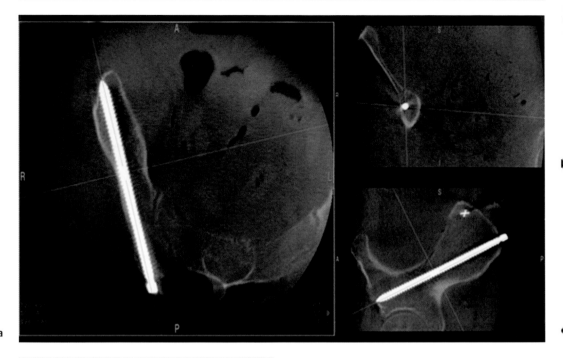

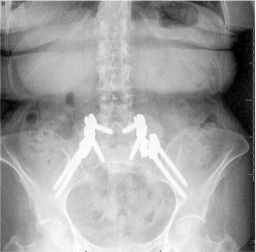

Fig. 4.2a–d Iliac screw placement using intraoperative computed tomography (CT)-based frameless navigation. **(a)** Iliac screw insertion point is at the posterior superior iliac spine, directed toward the anterior inferior iliac spine. **(b)** The teardrop view is utilized to optimize screw purchase in the lateral cortical wall, just above the sciatic notch. **(c)** The sagittal view is used to demonstrate screw angulation toward the anterior inferior iliac spine, avoiding violation of the acetabulum. **(d)** Stacked iliac screw construct in patient with progressive deformity from high-grade spondylolisthesis previously fused in situ, requiring sacral osteotomy for deformity correction.

screws, interbody cage, and iliac screws. Iliac screw or interbody cage placement significantly reduced multidirectional flexibility at the lumbosacral junction compared with pedicle screws alone, but iliac screw fixation was superior in protecting sacral screws from pullout or plowthrough.[4]

Lebwohl et al[5] performed a laboratory biomechanical analysis comparing construct stiffness, S1 screw strain, and ultimate failure load among several techniques of supplementary sacral fixation, using S1 pedicle screws with and without S2 screws, as well as an intrasacral rod and iliac screws. All techniques decreased the S1 screw strain in flexion-extension, but only iliac screws decreased S1 screw strain in axial loading. In destructive testing with flexion loading, only iliac screws significantly increased the load to failure. The authors concluded that the addition of iliac fixation significantly increases the biomechanical strength of sacral constructs.

A significant disadvantage to iliac screws is the potential prominence of the screw head at the posterior superior iliac spine (PSIS). Although the starting point can be modified or the PSIS notched to allow burying of the screw head, implant prominence cannot be completely eliminated. Another disadvantage is the requirement of an offset connector for segmental lumbosacral instrumentation.

Transsacral Iliac Fixation

S2-Alar-Iliac Screws

Developed to address the problematic implant prominence and offset location of iliac screws, S2-alar-iliac ("S2-iliac") screws are associated with a lower complication rate related to implant prominence-related pain, necessitating screw removal, compared with traditional iliac fixation.[11] Implant prominence is minimized, with the mean distance of the insertion point to the skin 15 mm deeper for the S2-iliac technique compared with traditional iliac screw insertion at the PSIS.[18] The S2-iliac screw starting point is 2 to 4 mm lateral and 4 to 8 mm caudal to the dorsal S1 foramen, with a trajectory toward the anterior inferior iliac spine (**Fig. 4.3a**) at an angle of ~ 40 degrees lateral and 20 to 30 degrees caudal.[11,18] The iliac teardrop is again employed for trajectory alignment. Unlike traditional iliac screws, S2-iliac screws do not typically require an offset connector for joining rods to lumbosacral pedicle screw constructs (**Fig. 4.3b**). Biomechanical testing of S2-iliac screws has shown equivalent stability to conventional iliac screws.[19] The S2-iliac screw trajectory results in crossing the sacroiliac joint, which has not been shown to be problematic in the first 5 years of follow-up of this technique, but which requires ongoing surveillance (**Fig. 4.3c,d**). Although haloing around iliac screws may be observed in over 25% of patients, iliac screw pullout or breakage is very rare.[1,11,14]

Adjunctive Anterior Interbody Support

Polly and colleagues[20] found that load-bearing interbody structural grafts increase construct stiffness and therefore can decrease the strain on posterior instrumentation, in addition to increasing the surface area available for arthrodesis. They also found that the location of the interbody graft in the sagittal plane has biomechanical significance, with anteriorly placed grafts having increased stiffness compared with central or posteriorly placed interbody grafts. Compared with stand-alone pedicle screw and combination pedicle-iliac screw constructs, pedicle-iliac screw constructs combined with interbody cages significantly reduce segmental movement across the lumbosacral junction in laboratory analysis.[4]

■ Patient Positioning

Patients undergoing sacral-pelvic instrumentation via open or minimally invasive technique should be positioned prone on an operating table that enables the creation or maintenance of anatomic lumbar lordosis. Fixation of the lumbosacral junction in a flat or kyphotic angulation must be absolutely avoided due to the resultant sagittal imbalance. Allowing the abdomen to hang freely without ventral compression helps minimize intra-abdominal pressure and venous bleeding.

■ Operative Techniques

Sacral Fixation

Pedicle screw pullout strength is increased by medialization of insertion trajectory compared with "straight-ahead" insertion without medial angulation of the screw tip.[3,12] An obese body habitus, an iliac crest overhang, or triangulated vertebral bodies may present obstacles to adequate medialization of pedicle screw trajectory (**Fig. 4.4a**). If this problem is encountered

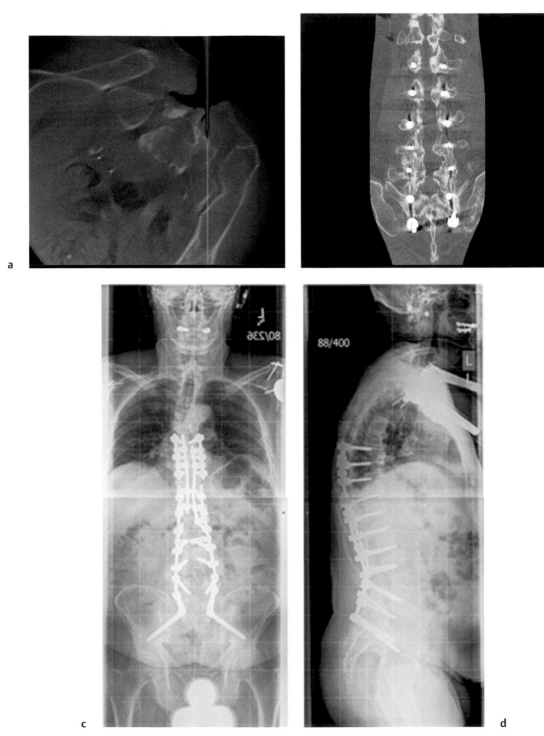

Fig. 4.3a–d S2-alar-iliac screws. **(a)** Intraoperative CT-guided planning demonstrating starting point and trajectory of S2-alar-iliac screw. **(b)** Postoperative CT scan showing alignment of S2-alar-iliac screw head with lumbosacral pedicle screws, eliminating the need for an offset connector typically required by traditional iliac screws. **(c,d)** X-rays demonstrating usage of S2-alar-iliac screws to anchor long construct for deformity correction.

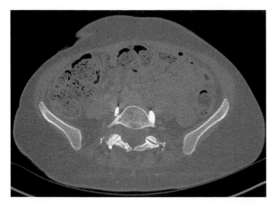

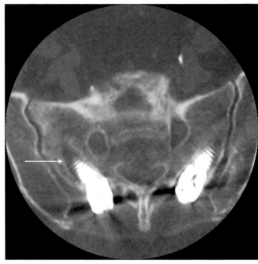

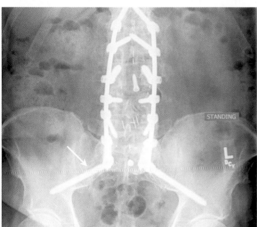

Fig. 4.4a–c Complications of sacral-pelvic fixation. **(a)** Failure to adequately direct pedicle screws in medial trajectory, combined with significant screw perforation of anterior cortex, resulting in screws abutting internal iliac veins bilaterally. **(b,c)** Asymptomatic halo formation (*arrows; dotted line*) around iliac screws does not necessitate revision unless resulting in pain or lumbosacral pseudarthrosis.

while using a midline open skin incision, the bailout technique requires splitting the fascia in a paramedian fashion for a transmuscular approach to enable a more lateral starting point and medialization of the trajectory. Vigilance is required to prevent an unintended straight-ahead trajectory from violating the anterior sacral or lumbar cortex with resultant injury to neurovascular structures. The aortic bifurcation occurs at approximately L4/L5, with the common iliac vessels traveling laterally from the bifurcation. The L4 and L5 nerve roots traverse the anterolateral sacral cortex prior to joining the lumbosacral plexus located at the level of the sacral ala, and the colon is in close opposition to the ventral surface of S2. A relative "safe zone" exists in the ventral midline of the sacral promontory; however, individual patient vascular anatomy should be incidentally visualized and appreciated on preoperative spine imaging prior to proceeding with instrumentation.

Iliac Fixation

Misdirection of iliac or S2-iliac screws through the sciatic notch can cause injury to the superior gluteal artery or sciatic nerve, which is a rare but serious complication. Violation of the acetabulum must be avoided. Familiarization with the iliac teardrop view enables correct screw trajectory selection.

Placement of screws into the ilium requires significant insertional torque that can cause breakage of the screwdriver unless care is taken to sequentially tap the screw trajectory completely to the desired depth. Once iliac screw insertion is initiated, one should not pause during insertion, as the mechanical thermal energy generated by screw insertion in the bone assists in temporarily lessening insertional torque, a benefit that is lost when screw insertion pauses. Iliac screw head prominence and offset distance from lumbosacral pedicle screw heads is minimized utilizing the S2-alar-iliac trajectory.

Revision of Screws

As mentioned, iliac screws may undergo asymptomatic haloing (**Fig. 4.4b,c**). Unless pain, implant breakage, or instability of the construct occurs, screw revision is not required. If iliac screw replacement is required, using larger diameter screws confers more stability than using longer screws.

■ Chapter Summary

Sacral-pelvic fixation is a powerful tool for increasing the strength and stability of lumbosacral constructs. Extreme biomechanical forces at the lumbosacral junction and relatively poor bone quality of the sacrum result in a high rate of lumbosacral pseudarthrosis and implant failure in adult spinal deformity correction. Sacral-pelvic fixation is indicated for lumbosacral arthrodesis extending cephalad to the L2 vertebra, augmentation of constructs for poor-quality or osteoporotic bone, sacrectomy for tumor or infection, unstable sacral fractures, correction of flat-back syndrome via lumbar osteotomy, correction of pelvic obliquity, high-grade spondylolisthesis, or as a salvage mechanism during revision for pseudarthrosis.

Sacral fixation is optimally performed using bi- or tricortical S1 medially directed pedicle screws. Alar and S2 screws and hooks through the dorsal sacral foramina may be added for supplementation, but lack the biomechanical strength to anchor long constructs in adult spinal deformity. Care must be taken to optimize screw size for cortical purchase while avoiding injury to neurovascular structures anterior to the lumbosacral junction.

Iliac fixation is optimally performed using iliac or S2-alar-iliac threaded screws, in a trajectory toward the anteroinferior iliac spine, with length ≥ 80 mm and diameter ≥ 9.5 mm. Knowledge of sacral-pelvic anatomy and use of the iliac teardrop view on intraoperative imaging is key for iliac screw placement.

The addition of interbody structural grafts increases the surface area for arthrodesis and stiffness of the construct and should be performed for long constructs at the lumbosacral junction.

The spinal deformity surgeon must have excellent knowledge of indications, instrumentation options, and techniques of sacral-pelvic fixation. Familiarization with sacral-pelvic anatomy is necessary to optimize the size and trajectory of instrumentation and avoid complications.

Pearls

- Sacral-pelvic fixation increases the strength and rigidity of constructs spanning the lumbosacral junction.
- Iliac fixation decreases the rate of sacral instrumentation failure and reduces the incidence of lumbosacral pseudarthrosis.
- S2-alar-iliac screws provide strong biomechanical fixation, minimal implant prominence, and favorable implant alignment with lumbosacral pedicle screws for ease of rod contouring.

Pitfalls

- Sacral pedicle and alar screws have inadequate strength to anchor constructs extending cephalad to L2, predisposing the patient to lumbosacral pseudarthrosis unless sacral-pelvic fixation strategies are employed.
- Acetabular joint impingement or sciatic notch violation with resultant neurovascular injury can occur during placement of iliac screws unless intraoperative imaging with teardrop view is used.

References

Five Must-Read References

1. Kim YJ, Bridwell KH, Lenke LG, Cho KJ, Edwards CC II, Rinella AS. Pseudarthrosis in adult spinal deformity following multisegmental instrumentation and arthrodesis. J Bone Joint Surg Am 2006;88:721–728
2. Kostuik JP. Treatment of scoliosis in the adult thoracolumbar spine with special reference to fusion to the sacrum. Orthop Clin North Am 1988;19:371–381
3. Santos ER, Rosner MK, Perra JH, Polly DW Jr. Spinopelvic fixation in deformity: a review. Neurosurg Clin N Am 2007;18:373–384
4. Cunningham BW, Lewis SJ, Long J, Dmitriev AE, Linville DA, Bridwell KH. Biomechanical evaluation of lumbosacral reconstruction techniques for spondylolisthesis: an in vitro porcine model. Spine 2002; 27:2321–2327
5. Lebwohl NH, Cunningham BW, Dmitriev A, et al. Biomechanical comparison of lumbosacral fixation techniques in a calf spine model. Spine 2002;27: 2312–2320
6. McCord DH, Cunningham BW, Shono Y, Myers JJ, McAfee PC. Biomechanical analysis of lumbosacral fixation. Spine 1992;17(8, Suppl):S235–S243
7. Kim YJ, Bridwell KH, Lenke LG, Rinella AS, Edwards C II. Pseudarthrosis in primary fusions for adult idiopathic scoliosis: incidence, risk factors, and outcome analysis. Spine 2005;30:468–474
8. Moshirfar A, Rand FF, Sponseller PD, et al. Pelvic fixation in spine surgery. Historical overview, indications, biomechanical relevance, and current techniques. J Bone Joint Surg Am 2005;87(Suppl 2):89–106
9. Luk KD, Chen L, Lu WW. A stronger bicortical sacral pedicle screw fixation through the S1 endplate: an in vitro cyclic loading and pull-out force evaluation. Spine 2005;30:525–529
10. Lehman RA Jr, Kuklo TR, Belmont PJ Jr, Andersen RC, Polly DW Jr. Advantage of pedicle screw fixation directed into the apex of the sacral promontory over bicortical fixation: a biomechanical analysis. Spine 2002;27:806–811
11. Kebaish KM. Sacropelvic fixation: techniques and complications. Spine 2010;35:2245–2251
12. Koller H, Zenner J, Hempfing A, Ferraris L, Meier O. Reinforcement of lumbosacral instrumentation using S1-pedicle screws combined with S2-alar screws. Oper Orthop Traumatol 2013;25:294–314
13. Cunningham BW, Polly DW Jr. The use of interbody cage devices for spinal deformity: a biomechanical perspective. Clin Orthop Relat Res 2002;394:73–83
14. Tsuchiya K, Bridwell KH, Kuklo TR, Lenke LG, Baldus C. Minimum 5-year analysis of L5-S1 fusion using sacropelvic fixation (bilateral S1 and iliac screws) for spinal deformity. Spine 2006;31:303–308
15. Santos ER, Sembrano JN, Mueller B, Polly DW. Optimizing iliac screw fixation: a biomechanical study on screw length, trajectory, and diameter. J Neurosurg Spine 2011;14:219–225
16. Peelle MW, Lenke LG, Bridwell KH, Sides B. Comparison of pelvic fixation techniques in neuromuscular spinal deformity correction: Galveston rod versus iliac and lumbosacral screws. Spine 2006;31:2392–2398, discussion 2399
17. Tis JE, Helgeson M, Lehman RA, Dmitriev AE. A biomechanical comparison of different types of lumbopelvic fixation. Spine 2009;34:E866–E872
18. Chang TL, Sponseller PD, Kebaish KM, Fishman EK. Low profile pelvic fixation: anatomic parameters for sacral alar-iliac fixation versus traditional iliac fixation. Spine 2009;34:436–440
19. O'Brien JR, Yu W, Kaufman BE, et al. Biomechanical evaluation of S2 alar-iliac screws: effect of length and quad-cortical purchase as compared with iliac fixation. Spine 2013;38:E1250–E1255
20. Polly DW Jr, Klemme WR, Cunningham BW, Burnette JB, Haggerty CJ, Oda I. The biomechanical significance of anterior column support in a simulated single-level spinal fusion. J Spinal Disord 2000;13:58–62

5

Instrumentation Strategies in Osteoporotic Spine: How to Prevent Failure?

Ahmet Alanay and Caglar Yilgor

■ Introduction

Osteoporosis is an imbalance between bone formation and resorption that primarily affects trabecular bone. Progressive bone mineral loss and concomitant bony architecture changes result in pain, deformity, increased risk of fracture, and possible neural compression.

The spine is the most common site of osteoporotic fractures. Although most patients with acute vertebral compression fractures improve regardless of the treatment applied, no patient experiences spontaneous restoration of the vertebral height and achieves a realigned spine. Therefore, spinal instrumentation is eventually required for some patients.

With aging comes a higher incidence of comorbidities that further complicates the management of osteoporotic spine. The elderly today have more active lifestyles than did the elderly of previous generations, and they refuse to accept disability and deformity as a part of the aging process. Modifiable conditions such as pulmonary, coronary, and cerebrovascular disease and diabetes mellitus should be addressed in collaboration with the consulting medical and anesthesiology specialists to minimize the surgical risk and optimize the outcome. Patients who smoke, have a nutritional deficiency, are depressed, or are subject to other life stressors should be counseled preoperatively to reduce the impact of these factors.

Performing adult spinal reconstruction in patients with osteopenia requires careful preoperative planning, as osteopenia has impact on both idiopathic and degenerative disorders. Similarly, careful preoperative planning is required when performing a reconstruction on younger patients with secondary osteoporosis due to factors such as hypercortisolism, hyperthyroidism, hyperparathyroidism, alcohol abuse, and immobilization.

In patients with low bone mineral density (BMD), spinal implants cannot be placed as securely as in patients with normal BMD, and thus application of corrective forces through the weak bone–implant interface is difficult. To avoid failure in such situations, it is important to understand the biomechanics of the osteoporotic spine and to recognize that osteoporosis is a systemic disease. The main surgical goal should be set to treat the symptoms. This chapter discusses the pre- and postoperative measures that can be taken in treating patients with osteoporosis, and the surgical strategies that can be used to reduce the risk of failure.

■ Understanding the Modes of Failure in Osteoporotic Spine

In the osteoporotic spine, the two most common surgical problems are failure of the fixation or of the bone–implant interface, and adjacent segment failure, either of which may result in pseudarthrosis.

In the early postoperative period, pedicle and adjacent vertebral fractures are the most common failures, whereas in the late phase, pseudarthrosis with instrumentation failure, adjacent disk degeneration, and late compression fractures with progressive kyphosis occur more frequently.

Because the osteoporotic spine is less able to withstand force, even the stresses and strains that are entailed in the activities of daily living can cause postoperative implant failure, which may present as a sudden pain, a neurologic problem, or implant prominence.

Fixation Failure

Because the elastic modulus of the bone is smaller than that of the implant, and because the force transmissions follow the path of least resistance, the bone surrounding the screws fails before the implant does. This phenomenon is called screw toggling, and, under repetitive cycling loading, pedicle screws typically fail by cephalocaudal toggling. Then loosening and eventually pullout occur, stripping or fracturing the pedicle. The thinner lateral wall of the pedicle is more often fractured than the medial wall. The packing of a stripped screw hole with corticocancellous graft does not usually augment the pullout strength of osteoporotic pedicles, which is a possible salvage method in healthy bone.[1]

In a cement-augmented pedicle, the screw can be pulled out alone, causing no damage to the bone or the cement, or the screw and the cement can be pulled out together, creating either an enlarged hole in the pedicle or a pedicle fracture.

The dorsal lamina has a thicker cortical shell than does the ventral aspect, which contributes to its success in the osteoporotic spine. The main failure mechanism of the laminar hooks is lamina breakout, breaking the "ring" formed by the lamina, posterior vertebral body, and medial pedicle walls.

Fracture of the upper-instrumented vertebra is another commonly seen failure in the osteoporotic spine.

Adjacent Segment Problems

After fixation of the osteoporotic spine, almost 80% of the proximal junctional kyphosis occurs due to adjacent vertebra fractures.[2] Instability and adjacent disk degeneration are other possible mechanisms of adjacent segment failure.

The preoperative status of the adjacent segment and disk is the greatest predictor of the development of postoperative adjacent segment failure. One must avoid ending a fusion adjacent to a severely degenerated disk or to a segment with fixed obliquity or subluxation.

Nonunion and Pseudarthrosis

Similar to a healthy bone, an osteoporotic bone is also subject to pseudarthrosis, especially in fusions extending to the sacrum. Known risk factors include thoracolumbar kyphosis, positive sagittal balance greater than 5 cm, presence of hip osteoarthritis, and incomplete sacropelvic fixation.

■ Preoperative Measures

Quantifying Bone Quality

Grading scales from X-rays, dual-energy X-ray absorptiometry (DEXA), quantitative computed tomography (QCT), and microdensitometry can be used to diagnose and quantify osteoporosis in an adult surgical candidate. QCT provides separate BMD estimates of trabecular and cortical bone, and has a higher sensitivity due to its imaging in a cross-sectional plane. Although QCT is useful in predicting the fracture risk, there is no clear consensus on a correlation between the quantity of osteoporosis and the type of strategies that should be applied.

The DEXA values acquired from the femoral neck should be interpreted with caution because the bone density in the spine decreases earlier than in other skeletal sites in the early postmenopausal years due to turnover in this highly trabecular bone. Bone density at various skeletal sites begins to coincide at about age 70. Also, DEXA acquired from the vertebrae may be falsely elevated due to degenerative changes.

Therefore, the surgeon must be ready to deal with a weak bone regardless of the preoperative DEXA values.

Medical Treatment

It is well documented in the literature that BMD correlates with implant pullout strength. Therefore, preoperative medical treatment with bisphosphonates, recombinant parathyroid hormone (rPTH), calcitonin, selective estrogen receptor modulators, calcium, or vitamin D should be considered. It is also important to determine whether the benefit of medical treatment is sufficient enough to offset the delay in surgical treatment.

The choice, timing, and duration of postoperative pharmacological treatment for osteoporosis also remain controversial because these drugs may interfere with bone healing.

■ Intraoperative Measures

The loss of the quantity as well as the architecture of the osteoporotic bone may increase the risk of spinal surgery or make the surgical goals difficult to achieve. In these situations, specific pedicle screw characteristics and insertion techniques can be adopted, and surgical strategies such as addressing the pathomorphology of the osteoporotic vertebrae, handling soft tissue meticulously, enhancing anchor points, applying prophylactic vertebroplasty, using interbody support, and protecting the bone–implant interface are utilized to improve the rate of successful fixation. These techniques and strategies are discussed in the following subsections.

Pathomorphology of the Osteoporotic Vertebrae

It is well established that the bone quality varies in different parts of the vertebrae. The vertebral body itself is the most affected part of the osteoporotic vertebrae. The lamina, on the other hand, which is predominantly cortical, is rela-

tively spared and is potentially a stronger anchor. The morphometry of the pedicles are variable. This pattern of bone loss causes the pedicle screw fixation to be less effective in the osteoporotic bone. The fixation of the pedicle screws is achieved either by taking advantage of the relatively stronger cortical bone within the pedicle by increasing the screw diameter and avoiding tapping the screw path, or by augmenting the pedicle screw in various ways. Sublaminar fixation with wires, cables, hooks, and bands is also a good alternative because the lamina is less affected by osteoporosis.

The BMD also varies in different regions of the sacrum. Medial side has a higher BMD than the lateral side, and the superior sacral end plate has the highest. The screws should therefore be directed medially in a triangular fashion and toward the sacral promontory.

The T2 pedicle is generally stronger than T3–T6 pedicles, making T2 a good option for screw fixation or pedicle hooks as a strong upper anchor point.[3]

Pedicle Screw Factors

No consensus has yet been reached on the optimal screw diameter, length, and shape for fixation in the osteoporotic bone. However, several pedicle screw characteristics, together with the hole preparation and screw insertion tactics, are shown to achieve a better fixation and prevent implant failure.

Pedicle Screw Characteristics

Double-threaded pedicle screws have a cancellous threaded tip followed by a cortical thread. The wider pitch of cancellous thread provides additional grip in the cancellous bone, and the screw advances faster with higher insertion torque. The cortical thread in the pedicle area provides higher grip and less toggle due to denser threads.[4]

Conical (tapered) screws also increase insertional torque, but they cannot be reversed or backed out, because doing so eradicates the screw's contact with the bone.

The expandable pedicle screw uses a novel screw design that enables the distal part of the screw to enlarge within the vertebral body as a posteriorly directed force is applied to the screw to resist pullout failure. The tip of the screw becomes anchored against the inner cortex of the dorsal vertebral body, resulting in a 76% increase in holding strength in comparison to conventional pedicle screws,[5] by taking advantage of the relatively uncompromised cortical bone rather than depending solely on weakened osteoporotic cancellous bone. However, in patients with severely low BMD, expandable screws may be unable to overcome the extreme biomechanical disadvantage, resulting in failure. Moreover, screw revision remains an issue in the clinical application of these screws.

Pedicle Screw Tract Augmentation

It is possible to augment the pedicle screw tract by preparing the hole, injecting polymethylmethacrylate (PMMA) bone cement into the hole, and inserting the screw afterwards. Augmentation may also be done with bioactive cements, calcium phosphate, or calcium sulfate using traditional or fenestrated pedicle screws. Coating the pedicle screw with hydroxyapatite is a time-dependent augmentation technique that increases osteointegration.

Cement Augmentation and Fenestrated Screws

A cadaveric biomechanical analysis of PMMA-augmented pedicle screw fixation using a novel fenestrated bone tap increased the pullout strength by 199% and 162% in primary and revision procedures, respectively.[6] Clinical series also demonstrated good outcome with no screw loosening, migration, or pullout detected in the follow-up X-rays, no fracture at the augmented levels, and no implant failure requiring reintervention.[7,8]

Although PMMA augmentation of the pedicle screws provides good fixation in patients with low BMD, it is not free of complications. Extravasation, intracanal leakage, hypotension, increase in pulmonary artery pressure, pulmonary cement emboli, superficial infections, and thermal nerve injuries were reported. Therefore, strategies were developed to reduce the

likelihood of cement leakage. Higher viscosity cement can be used, and fluoroscopy can provide additional assistance. It is generally recommended to inject 1 to 3 mL of cement because using a larger amount fails to demonstrate any significant benefit in pullout strength.[6]

Attention was also paid to the method of PMMA augmentation. Injecting cement into a cavity prepared by an inflatable balloon followed by insertion of the pedicle screw demonstrated almost twice the pullout strength of screws augmented with standard cement injection.[9] Fenestrated screws have been used more recently, with promising results.[10] Although clinical long-term results are yet to be seen, there is a potential theoretical advantage of using fenestrated screws over injecting cement followed by screw insertion. Injecting the cement into the prepared hole fills the tract, and when inserting the pedicle screw, the cement coats the screw threads and thereby reduces effective screw purchase. Alternatively, cement injection through a fenestrated screw enables the cement to infiltrate in the vertebral body without altering the bone–implant interface.[11]

Although it is widely used with promising results, PMMA is toxic, is unable to undergo remodeling after microfracture within the cement, and is difficult to remove in revision surgery. Hence, osteobiologic cement is an area of interest and development for screw augmentation. Calcium phosphate and calcium sulfate avoid the exothermic reaction and reduce the risk of leakage. Moreover, they are bioresorbable and potentially osteoconductive, and integrate in the natural process of bony remodeling. A cadaveric study comparing osteobiologic cement and PMMA for the use of screw augmentation found no significant differences in axial pullout strength.[12]

Hydroxyapatite Coating

The increased osteointegration of the hydroxyapatite-coated pedicle screws is time dependent; with time, optimum stability is achieved. It has been shown in an osteoporotic animal model that hydroxyapatite-coated pedicle screws are 1.6 times more resistant to pullout and that they have superior biological bonding to the surrounding bone, occurring as early as 10 days after surgery.[13] However, they do not allow for the application of additional forces during intraoperative correction maneuvers.

Insertion Technique and Insertional Torque

The starting point, hole preparation, tapping, the insertion angle, and the trajectory of a pedicle screw, as well as its length, depth of penetration, and diameter, affect its insertional torque and thereby its resistance to failure.

Length of Screw and Depth of Screw Penetration

The length of a pedicle screw is linearly related to its pullout strength. As the screw penetrates further into the vertebral body, the cutout load to failure increases. By engaging the ventral cortex of the vertebral body, screws can be placed in a bicortical fashion to provide up to an additional 30% of pullout strength.[14] The risk–benefit ratio should be considered, and care must be taken to avoid injury to adjacent structures when using this technique.

Diameter

The diameter of the pedicle screw should be as wide as possible to enable better cortical bone purchase. Increasing the diameter increases the pullout strength in milder cases; however, in severe osteoporosis the pullout force is low regardless of the screw diameter. Instead, using larger diameters may cause dilation or fracture of the pedicle that decreases its strength.[15]

Starting Point, Insertion Angle, and Trajectory

When the screws are placed parallel, the volume of cancellous bone between the threads of the screw determines the resistance to pullout for each screw. Triangulated screws provide better pullout strength with a larger volume of cancellous bone available for resistance to pullout because the construct is contributed by the volume of bone within the trapezoid area in the vertebral body formed by longer and triangulated screws.[16]

Thoracic Spine

In the anatomic trajectory, the screw is in line with the pedicle axis and therefore is directed to the inferior corner of the vertebral body in the sagittal plane. In the straightforward technique, the screw is parallel to the vertebral end plate and triangulation in the transverse plane can be achieved. This technique provides at least 39% higher maximum insertional torque and 27% greater pullout strength.[17] Pedicle-rib screws increase the effective transverse diameter when compared with the pedicle alone and can be used for safer insertion of the screws, although it may decrease the pullout strength by 25%.[18] The starting point should be selected in accordance with the trajectory used.

Lumbar Spine

Placing the pedicle screws in convergence also increases the pullout strength in the lumbar spine.

Sacrum and Pelvis

Sacral fixation is a big challenge in the osteoporotic spine. Restoration of the sagittal balance is more important than the fixation itself.

When the fusion is extended to the sacrum and a long fusion is performed, multiple and bicortical screw fixation should be used in addition to consideration of anterior column support or iliac fixation. The tricortical technique, which entails directing the screws into the sacral promontory, increases the insertional torque.[19]

Hole Preparation and Tapping

Appropriate preparation of the hole improves screw purchase. High insertional torque improves the screw pullout strength. In healthy vertebral bodies, the screws are placed after tapping to avoid microfracturing within the dense bony matrix of the bone during screw insertion. In osteoporotic cancellous bone, however, tapping results in removal of bone within the pedicle track and prevents bone compression around the screw threads. Even screw removal and immediate reinsertion decreases the mechanical insertion torque. Therefore, under-tapping or not tapping at all is advised in osteoporotic bone. When compared with same-size tapping, under-tapping by 0.5 and 1.0 mm increases the insertional torque by 47% and 93%, respectively.[20]

Under-tapping is more beneficial in the lumbar spine than in the thoracic spine. This may be due to the fact that the thoracic pedicle screws are probably more dependent on cortical purchase within the pedicle walls.

Enhancing Anchor Points

The weak link in the osteoporotic spine instrumentation is the implant–bone interface. Fixation strategies for osteoporotic bone are targeted toward taking advantage of the relatively stronger cortical bone. Anchor options, in addition to screws, include hooks, wires, cables, and bands.

Load Sharing by Multilevel Fixation

Because the implant–bone interface in the osteoporotic bone is prone to failure, the number of points of fixation must be increased to distribute the contact forces more evenly. Longer constructs with at least three sets of fixation points at each end can be beneficial, keeping in mind the added morbidity entailed with using additional screws.

As previously stated, using hooks, wires, cables, and bands as well as cross-links help in improving the performance of the pedicle screws.

Selection of Fusion Levels

End-instrumented vertebrae should be carefully selected. Ending the construct in a kyphotic region or at the apex of kyphosis should be avoided.

Another frequent decision-making dilemma in the osteoporotic spine is whether or not to fuse to sacrum. Certain scenarios that require lumbosacral fixation are symptomatic L5-S1

spondylolisthesis, over 15 degrees of scoliosis at the L5-S1 segment, and the need to achieve proper sagittal balance.[21] Stopping at L5 entails the risk of increased adjacent segment disease, whereas fusing to the sacrum is found to have more complications.[21] L5 pedicles are usually short and contain more cancellous bone. Therefore, it may be risky to end a long fusion at L5 in osteoporotic patients because L5 pedicle screws may fail.

Cross-Link

The use of a rigid or semirigid cross-link, especially when the screws are triangulated, increases the torsional stiffness by making the construct perform effectively as a quadrilateral frame. The use of a cross-link is especially advantageous in longer constructs, as it prevents rods from telescoping.

Hooks, Wires, Cables, and Bands

The use of sublaminar and pediculolaminar hooks, wires, cables, and bands takes advantage of the cortical bone composition of the spinal lamina.

A polyester band may be used to increase the surface of bony contact and to fit any anatomy. It may be used in a sublaminar, subpars, transversal, or laminotransversal fashion to enable translation, distraction and compression, in situ bending, and rod derotation.

Prophylactic Vertebroplasty

In the setting of osteoporosis, junctional failure, especially in the cranial levels, is not a rare occurrence. Prevention is the best way to overcome adjacent segment failure. Prophylactic vertebroplasty entails cement augmentation of the adjacent noninstrumented segment/segments. Although there is a paucity of clinical and biomechanical studies, prophylactic vertebroplasty seems to be helpful in decreasing the revision arthrodesis rates because of adjacent vertebrae fractures.[22]

Further studies are needed to clarify the optimum amount of cement required and how many levels should be prophylactically cemented. Efficacy at the distal adjacent level also needs to be further analyzed.

Interbody Support in Osteoporotic Spine

Anterior column support is beneficial in load sharing because the graft or cage lessens the stress directed toward the screw–rod construct. Anterior interbody support may further improve sagittal spinal balance and rates of arthrodesis.

Interbody grafts serve a more critical role at the caudal end of the construct, particularly at the lumbosacral junction. Grafts can be placed with a bias toward the concavity of the deformity to assist correction. **Figs. 5.1, 5.2,** and **5.3**

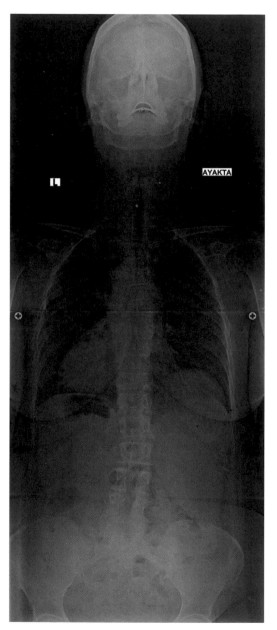
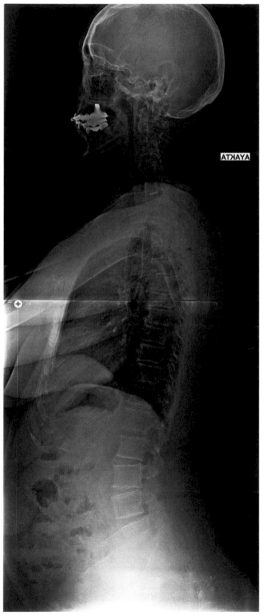

a
b

Fig. 5.1a,b **(a)** Preoperative posteroanterior X-ray. **(b)** Preoperative lateral X-ray.

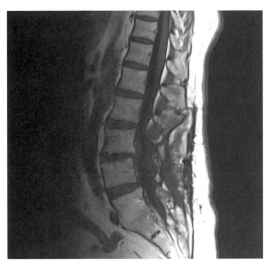
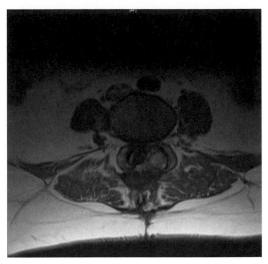

a   b

Fig. 5.2a,b (a) Preoperative sagittal magnetic resonance imaging (MRI) view. **(b)** Preoperative transverse MRI view.

demonstrate the use of the intraoperative measures mentioned above in a 64-year-old patient with a BMD of –3.2 complaining of back and leg pain.

In severe osteoporosis, there is a risk of subsidence of the graft or cage into the end plates that may lead to anterior column collapse and subsequent kyphotic deformity. The cage should be placed to contact the peripheral apophyseal ring where the cortical bone is stronger. A graft with an elastic modulus that is similar to the native bone also reduces the risk of subsidence. Choices of interbody graft materials include bone (autograft or allograft), metal, carbon fiber, polyaryletheretherketone (PEEK), and other synthetic materials. Iliac crest autograft is typically the best match, but it is associated with well-established harvest-related morbidity.

Role of Anterior Fixation in the Osteoporotic Spine

Continuous loading of anterior screw constructs on a low-BMD spine can lead to screw cutout. Although newer implant designs demonstrate improved anchorage,[23] anterior fixation has a limited role in the osteoporotic spine because it is the most affected part of the vertebrae.

Role of Semirigid Fixation in the Osteoporotic Spine

The loading of the spine in various axes of motion creates increased stress at the bone–implant interface. The difference of the rigidity within the instrumented and noninstrumented segments of the spine can accelerate adjacent segment degeneration and potentially cause pseudarthrosis. Semirigid fixation may provide sufficient stabilization to facilitate bony fusion while permitting some degree of flexibility to offload stress at the adjacent segment and the bone–implant interface.

Protection of the Bone–Implant Interface

Handling intraoperative soft tissue meticulously, providing extensive release, performing osteotomies to increase flexibility and thus minimize the corrective forces, maintaining sagittal alignment, and obtaining a solid fusion are essential for the protection of the bone–implant interface.

Meticulous Soft Tissue Handling

Care should be taken to preserve the supraspinous ligament, intraspinous ligament, and

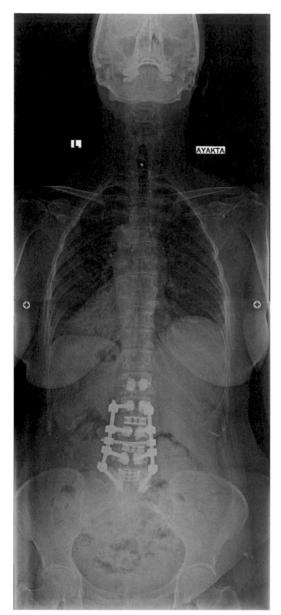

a

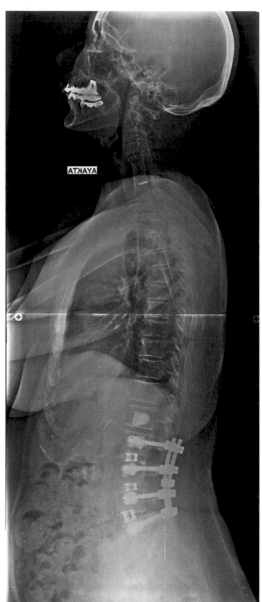

b

Fig. 5.3a,b (a) Last follow-up posteroanterior X-ray of the same patient demonstrating the use of cement-augmented pedicle screws, anterior interbody support, prophylactic vertebroplasty, and cross-link. **(b)** Last follow-up lateral X-ray of the same patient demonstrating the use of cement-augmented pedicle screws, anterior interbody support, prophylactic vertebroplasty, and cross-link.

ligamentum flavum between the cranial fused level and the adjacent segment, as well as between the cranial levels of fusion. Doing so provides a segment of higher posterior tension, which may prevent the development of junctional deformity and instability. Supra- and infra-adjacent facets should be preserved and the cranial disk space should not be violated with pedicle screws.

Extensive Release

The release of the diskoligamentous and bony constraints such as diskectomy, facetectomy, or various osteotomies should be optimized before reductionto decrease the stress applied to the bone–implant interface when performing spinal corrective maneuvers.

Maintaining Sagittal Alignment

Aligning the osteoporotic spine to physiological coronal and sagittal contours neutralizes the deforming forces, reduces the junctional forces, and decreases the energy required for ambulation.

Obtaining Fusion

Obtaining a rapid and solid fusion ensures long-term spinal stability, reducing the load on instruments and on the relatively poor bone–implant interface. A thorough fusion procedure with appropriate bone-bed preparation and appropriate use of bone grafts or substitutes is therefore of particular importance in the osteoporotic spine. The use of bone morphogenetic protein may facilitate an earlier and more vigorous fusion, and decrease the risk of implant-related failure. The use of bone morphogenetic protein may also be associated with complications related to soft tissue swelling, inappropriate bone formation around neural elements, and subsequent radiculitis.

■ Postoperative Measures

Enhancing the purchase of internal fixation and protecting the bone–implant interface by han-

dling soft tissue meticulously, providing extensive releases, maintaining sagittal alignment, and using anterior interbody support decreases the demand on fixation in the postoperative period. External brace immobilization and restriction of the spine range of motion as well as physical therapy and rehabilitation are measures that can be taken in the postoperative period to serve the same purpose. As stated earlier, the timing of postoperative pharmacological osteoporosis treatment remains controversial.

If a brace is to be used, it must be custom-molded postoperatively, after surgical deformity correction is established. Rehabilitation should focus on gait training, balance, and general conditioning, together with range-of-motion and flexibility exercises of the hip and knee. There is no consensus yet on the duration of brace application.

■ Chapter Summary

Primarily affecting the trabecular bone, osteoporosis causes progressive bone mineral loss and concomitant bony architecture changes that result in pain, deformity, increased fracture risk, and possible neural compression. Although most patients with acute, painful vertebral compression fractures improve regardless of the treatment applied, no patient spontaneously restores the vertebral height and achieves a realigned spine. Spinal instrumentation is eventually required in some osteoporotic patients. In the setting of osteoporosis, however, the fixation of the spinal implants is insecure, and application of corrective forces through a weak bone–implant interface is difficult, complicating the surgical treatment. The first step for an adult spinal surgical candidate is the diagnosis and quantification of the osteoporosis. Understanding the biomechanics and the modes of failure of the osteoporotic spine is important. The vertebral body itself is the most affected part of the osteoporotic vertebrae. The lamina, on the other hand, which is predominantly cortical, is relatively spared and is potentially a stronger anchor. The morphometry of the pedicles is variable. Failure of the fixation or of the bone–implant interface, adjacent segment failures, and pseudarthrosis are the three main problems in osteoporotic spine. Several pre- and postoperative measures may be taken, as well as applying several surgical strategies intraoperatively to prevent failure. The pedicle screw characteristics together with hole preparation and screw insertion tactics are shown to achieve a better fixation. Anterior column support is beneficial in load sharing, improving sagittal balance and reducing the rates of arthrodesis. The results of cement augmentation of the pedicle screws and the adjacent noninstrumented vertebrae seem promising, but it is not a complication-free procedure.

Pearls

◆ In elective cases, increasing the BMD preoperatively with parathyroid hormone might be considered.
◆ Under-tapping is advised in the osteoporotic bone to increase the insertional torque.
◆ Triangulated screws provide better pullout strength, with a larger volume of cancellous bone available for resistance to pullout because the construct is contributed by the volume of bone within the trapezoid area in the vertebral body formed by the longer and triangulated screws.
◆ The use of a cross-link is especially advantageous in longer constructs, as it prevents rods from telescoping.
◆ The use of hooks, wires, cables, and bands take advantage of the relatively stronger cortical bone for fixation of osteoporotic bone.

◆ Cement-augmented pedicle screws are advantageous for better fixation and for allowing additional corrective forces.
◆ Prophylactic vertebroplasty is helpful in decreasing the revision arthrodesis rates because of adjacent vertebrae fractures.
◆ The release of the diskoligamentous and bony constraints such as diskectomy, facetectomy, or various osteotomies should be optimized before reduction when performing spinal corrective procedures to decrease the stress applied to the bone–implant interface.
◆ A custom-molded postoperative brace helps protect the bone–implant interface.

Pitfalls

◆ Avoid ending a fusion adjacent to a severely degenerated disk or to a segment with fixed obliquity or subluxation.
◆ DEXA scans in elderly patients must be interpreted with caution because degenerative changes may falsely elevate the BMD values.
◆ In the osteoporotic bone, tapping results in removal of bone within the pedicle track and prevents bone compression around the screw threads.
◆ Avoid ending a construct in a kyphotic region or at the apex of kyphosis.
◆ Avoid damaging the supra- and intraspinous ligaments and ligamentum flavum between the cranial fused level and the adjacent segment, as well as between the cranial levels of fusion.
◆ Avoid damaging the supra- and infra-adjacent facets and violating the cranial disk space with pedicle screws.

References
Five Must-Read References
1. Halvorson TL, Kelley LA, Thomas KA, Whitecloud TS III, Cook SD. Effects of bone mineral density on pedicle screw fixation. Spine 1994;19:2415–2420
2. DeWald CJ, Stanley T. Instrumentation-related complications of multilevel fusions for adult spinal deformity patients over age 65: surgical considerations and treatment options in patients with poor bone quality. Spine 2006;31(19, Suppl):S144–S151
3. Butler TE Jr, Asher MA, Jayaraman G, Nunley PD, Robinson RG. The strength and stiffness of thoracic implant anchors in osteoporotic spines. Spine 1994;19:1956–1962
4. Mummaneni PV, Haddock SM, Liebschner MA, Keaveny TM, Rosenberg WS. Biomechanical evaluation of a double-threaded pedicle screw in elderly vertebrae. J Spinal Disord Tech 2002;15:64–68
5. McKoy BE, An YH. An expandable anchor for fixation in osteoporotic bone. J Orthop Res 2001;19:545–547
6. Frankel BM, D'Agostino S, Wang C. A biomechanical cadaveric analysis of polymethylmethacrylate-augmented pedicle screw fixation. J Neurosurg Spine 2007;7:47–53
7. Chang MC, Liu CL, Chen TH. Polymethylmethacrylate augmentation of pedicle screw for osteoporotic spi-

nal surgery: a novel technique. Spine 2008;33:E317–E324

8. Aydogan M, Ozturk C, Karatoprak O, Tezer M, Aksu N, Hamzaoglu A. The pedicle screw fixation with vertebroplasty augmentation in the surgical treatment of the severe osteoporotic spines. J Spinal Disord Tech 2009;22:444–447

9. Burval DJ, McLain RF, Milks R, Inceoglu S. Primary pedicle screw augmentation in osteoporotic lumbar vertebrae: biomechanical analysis of pedicle fixation strength. Spine 2007;32:1077–1083

10. Chang MC, Kao HC, Ying SH, Liu CL. Polymethylmethacrylate augmentation of cannulated pedicle screws for fixation in osteoporotic spines and comparison of its clinical results and biomechanical characteristics with the needle injection method. J Spinal Disord Tech 2013;26:305–315

11. Wang MY, Hoh DJ. Bone metabolism and osteoporosis and its effects on spinal disease and surgical treatments. In: Winn HR, ed. Youmans' Neurological Surgery. Philadelphia: Elsevier; 2011

12. Rohmiller MT, Schwalm D, Glattes RC, Elalayli TG, Spengler DM. Evaluation of calcium sulfate paste for augmentation of lumbar pedicle screw pullout strength. Spine J 2002;2:255–260

13. Hasegawa T, Inufusa A, Imai Y, Mikawa Y, Lim TH, An HS. Hydroxyapatite-coating of pedicle screws improves resistance against pull-out force in the osteoporotic canine lumbar spine model: a pilot study. Spine J 2005;5:239–243

14. Zindrick MR, Wiltse LL, Widell EH, et al. A biomechanical study of intrapeduncular screw fixation in the lumbosacral spine. Clin Orthop Relat Res 1986; 203:99–112

15. Yazici M, Pekmezci M, Cil A, Alanay A, Acaroglu E, Oner FC. The effect of pedicle expansion on pedicle morphology and biomechanical stability in the immature porcine spine. Spine 2006;31:E826–E829

16. Hadjipavlou AG, Nicodemus CL, al-Hamdan FA, Simmons JW, Pope MH. Correlation of bone equivalent mineral density to pull-out resistance of triangulated pedicle screw construct. J Spinal Disord 1997;10: 12–19

17. Lehman RA Jr, Polly DW Jr, Kuklo TR, Cunningham B, Kirk KL, Belmont PJ Jr. Straight-forward versus anatomic trajectory technique of thoracic pedicle screw fixation: a biomechanical analysis. Spine 2003;28: 2058–2065

18. White KK, Oka R, Mahar AT, Lowry A, Garfin SR. Pullout strength of thoracic pedicle screw instrumentation: comparison of the transpedicular and extrapedicular techniques. Spine 2006;31:E355–E358

19. Lehman RA Jr, Kuklo TR, Belmont PJ Jr, Andersen RC, Polly DW Jr. Advantage of pedicle screw fixation directed into the apex of the sacral promontory over bicortical fixation: a biomechanical analysis. Spine 2002;27:806–811

20. Kuklo TR, Lehman RA Jr. Effect of various tapping diameters on insertion of thoracic pedicle screws: a biomechanical analysis. Spine 2003;28:2066–2071

21. Bridwell KH, Edwards CC II, Lenke LG. The pros and cons to saving the L5-S1 motion segment in a long scoliosis fusion construct. Spine 2003;28:S234–S242

22. Chiang CK, Wang YH, Yang CY, Yang BD, Wang JL. Prophylactic vertebroplasty may reduce the risk of adjacent intact vertebra from fatigue injury: an ex vivo biomechanical study. Spine 2009;34:356–364

23. Goldhahn J, Reinhold M, Stauber M, et al. Improved anchorage in osteoporotic vertebrae with new implant designs. J Orthop Res 2006;24:917–925

6

The Incidence and Management of Acute Neurologic Complications Following Complex Adult Spinal Deformity Surgery

Joseph S. Butler and Lawrence G. Lenke

■ Introduction

Significant advances have been made in adult spinal deformity (ASD) surgery over the past several years. Improvements in pedicle screw technology and the increasing use of three-column osteotomies have made more powerful deformity corrections possible. Nonetheless, loss of neurologic function after ASD surgery remains a serious and potentially devastating complication, with profound consequences for health-related quality of life. Intraoperative neurophysiology monitoring has become a reliable and effective modality to optimize neurologic safety during ASD surgery.[1,2] Furthermore, the increasing use of image-guided navigation systems has led to significant improvements in the accuracy of pedicle screw placement.[3,4] This chapter discusses the management of acute neurologic complications in complex ASD surgery and proposes a treatment algorithm to deal with these complications in safe and effective manner.

■ Prevalence

The incidence of neurologic complications in ASD patients undergoing deformity correction surgery has been difficult to determine. Multiple flaws exist in the published data, with a lack of high-quality prospective studies, significant data variability, and a lack of rigorous and validated measurements of neurologic function. Nonetheless, the incidence of neurologic deficits following ASD surgery has been previously reported as ranging from 0% to over 10%.[5-9]

Two previous studies, one from a single institution, analyzed prospectively collected data to identify complications, but neither one used a validated scoring system to quantify neurologic function.[10,11] All studies could more accurately be described as retrospective studies of prospectively collected data. But an accurate rate of neurologic complications after complex ASD surgery is critical for informed decision making for both patients and surgeons. Furthermore, it is crucial to be able to measure changes in neurologic complication rates in a standardized fashion so as to accurately evaluate new techniques, technologies, and therapies in ASD surgery.

The Scoli-Risk-1 trial is a recent prospective, multicenter observational study attempting to accurately assess the neurologic complication rate following complex ASD surgery using the American Spinal Injury Association (ASIA) scoring system (**Fig. 6.1**).[12] A total of 276 patients

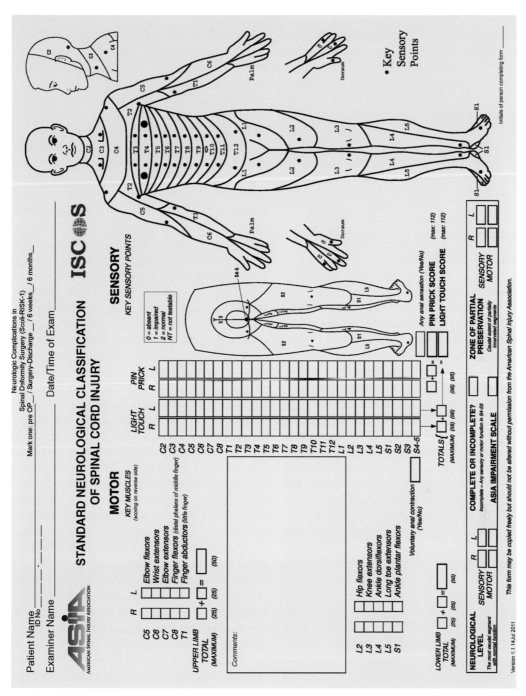

Fig. 6.1 The American Spinal Injury Association (ASIA) scoring system.

were enrolled from 15 international centers. At hospital discharge, 23.1% of patients had a measurable lower extremity motor deficit (i.e., less than 5/5 motor strength in all five major leg muscles) decreasing to 17.8% at 6 weeks and 10.7% at 6 months postoperative. This study gives a clearer indication of the expected neurologic complication rate in ASD patients, potentially setting a standard for future clinical trials aimed at lowering the rate of postoperative neurologic deficits.

■ Mechanisms of Neurologic Complications

There are several proposed causes of intraoperative neurologic deficits during ASD surgery. Intraoperative spinal cord, cauda equina, or nerve root deficits may result from direct neurologic trauma during instrumentation such as the placement of pedicle screws, hooks, or sublaminar wires. Furthermore, intraoperative corrective maneuvers may lead to neurologic deficit secondary to either distraction of the neural elements or excessive tension on local vasculature, leading to decreased blood flow and cord ischemia. Spinal cord ischemia may also result from prolonged extreme hypotension (mean arterial pressure [MAP] < 55 mm Hg), hypoxia secondary to decreased hemoglobin level, or vascular compromise after ligation of the segmental vessels in an anterior procedure.[13]

■ Patient Evaluation and Preoperative Planning

Neurologic complications are most strongly associated with prolonged complex surgery, a large amount of blood loss, combined anterior/posterior procedures, multistage surgery, congenital kyphosis or scoliosis, large or rigid spinal curves (Cobb angle > 90 degrees), preexisting myelopathy or neurologic deficit, and intramedullary spinal cord tumors. Further risk factors include tethered cord, Arnold-Chiari malformation, syringomyelia, and split cord malformations.

A complete patient history and thorough physical examination still remain essential elements to an adequate preoperative workup. Patients should be assessed for a history of congenital deformities such as kyphosis and scoliosis, neurofibromatosis, and skeletal dysplasia, which would infer a considerably increased risk of iatrogenic neurologic complications. The physical examination should include a three-dimensional assessment of the spine to evaluate patient posture, neurologic status, hip flexion contractures, leg length inequality, pelvic obliquity, body habitus, and nutritional status. Meticulous examination of the motor, sensory, and reflex function as well as gait assessment is critical in screening patients for potential intraspinal and brainstem anomalies such as tethered cord, Arnold-Chiari malformation, syringomyelia, and split cord malformations.

Adequate radiological imaging is crucial for optimal surgical and neurologic outcome. However, it is technique-dependent, requiring visualization of the entire spine in the coronal and sagittal planes, including the hip joints, with all imaging taken with the patient standing with the knees fully extended for accurate measurement of sagittal balance (sagittal vertical axis [SVA]), thoracic kyphosis, lumbar lordosis, and spinopelvic parameters including pelvic incidence (PI), sacral slope (SS), and pelvic tilt (PT). Lateral dynamic standing lumbar X-rays may identify focal instability or spondylolisthesis. Bending films and supine X-rays without the effects of gravity help assess the flexibility of a deformity. Once the appropriate radiographic studies have been obtained, the sagittal and coronal balance can then be assessed.

Magnetic resonance imaging (MRI) is used as a routine preoperative radiographic study to assess central canal stenosis, facet hypertrophy, pedicular anomaly, foraminal encroachment, and degenerative disk disease. It also helps determine the presence of intraspinal anomalies. Patients with suspected low bone mass or with established osteoporosis should have a dual-energy X-ray absorptiometry (DEXA) scan performed to optimize surgical planning.

■ Intraoperative Preparation

Meticulous intraoperative preparation is required for the safe and effective management of intraoperative complications. Before induction of anesthesia, the surgical team should discuss with the anesthesia and neuromonitoring teams and operating room staff the patient's medical situation, the intended procedure, and surgical time frame. An arterial line may be used to monitor MAP. Somatosensory evoked potential (SSEP) and motor evoked potential (MEP) leads are placed and checked before the patient is turned to the prone position. The upper extremities are padded and positioned to avoid stretch or compression of the brachial plexus, and care is taken to ensure that the pressure areas are well padded. Forced-air warming blankets prevent hypothermia, particularly in procedures of long duration.

Maintaining adequate blood pressure is essential. However, a balance should be maintained to minimize intraoperative blood loss and transfusions, yet ensuring adequate spinal cord perfusion. A MAP of < 55 mm Hg has been associated with an increased risk of spinal cord ischemia.[14] However, mild hypotensive anesthesia is often used to minimize blood loss, particularly during the surgical approach, with the MAP maintained at 65 to 70 mm Hg. Approximately 30 minutes before performing corrective maneuvers, the anesthesia team should gradually elevate the MAP to > 70–80 mm Hg to maintain adequate cord perfusion during spinal column manipulation and deformity correction.

■ Intraoperative Neuromonitoring

Stagnara Wake-Up Test

The Stagnara wake-up test has been widely used in the intraoperative assessment of neurologic function. It assesses primary motor cortex, anterior motor pathways of the spinal cord, nerve roots, and peripheral nerves. However, it gives only a gross approximation of the function of these elements and does not directly measure any components of the sensory system.[15] This test involves a temporary reduction in anesthesia, after which the patient is asked to move the upper and lower extremities. The test is limited, as it is entirely reliant on patient compliance and cannot be used in patients unable to follow commands because of intellectual and developmental disability, young age, or preoperative weakness. The test itself carries risk, including self-extubation, loss of intravenous access or of safe patient-positioning on the table, air embolism, and postoperative recollection of the event.

The wake-up test was historically the benchmark for intraoperative neurologic assessment, and is still used at some centers in conjunction with advanced neuromonitoring techniques as a means of confirming neurologic status. Properly administered, the wake-up test should be 100% accurate in detecting gross motor changes.[15] Although the limitations of the test prevent assessment of fine motor changes, it will alert the surgeon to the most clinically significant neurologic deficits. It is used when there is any problem obtaining spinal cord monitoring (SCM) signals (such as in a patient with thoracic myelopathy) and also in patient's who have had SCM changes meeting evoked potential warning criteria when the responses cannot be improved. It also should always be performed at the end of the surgical procedure prior to the patient's leaving the operating room.

Somatosensory Evoked Potentials

Somatosensory evoked potentials assess the posterior columns of the spinal cord, in addition to the cerebral cortex and mixed peripheral nerves. The posterior columns are responsible for proprioception as opposed to pain and temperature. Although proprioceptive loss is not as debilitating as a motor deficit, it can have a significant impact on activities of daily living. As SSEPs are sensitive to focal posterior column and global spinal cord issues, they act as a good surrogate for other neural pathways. However, there are situations when a motor deficit might not be demonstrated on SSEP monitoring. For example, anterior vascular territory compromise without concomitant posterior vascular changes might not be addressed by SSEP monitoring.

Somatosensory evoked potentials continue to be the most frequently used intraoperative monitoring method to assess the integrity of the dorsal column but cannot be relied on to monitor motor function directly. Reports of postoperative paraparesis in the absence of intraoperative SSEP signal change underscores this important limitation.[16] SSEP dependability falls off when applied to patients with preexisting neurologic conditions. Individual nerve root injury is not effectively monitored by SSEPs. Missed nerve root or isolated motor pathway complications are not failures of the modality but rather are issues outside of SSEP monitoring capability, highlighting the need for alternative or adjunct monitoring approaches. Warning criteria for SSEPs at out institution include greater than a 60% decrease in amplitude or a 10% increase in latency of the signal as compared with baseline values.

Motor Evoked Potentials

Motor evoked potentials monitor corticospinal tract activity via stimulation at the level of the motor cortex or spinal cord and are selective for motor pathways. MEP monitoring relies on intervening thalamic synapses to prevent antidromic firing of spinal sensory tracts. The stimulation site for transcranial MEP (tcMEP) is the cerebral cortex. MEP end-point data are ascertained from the spinal cord (D-wave) or from the end muscle compound motor action potential (CMAP). Stimuli are presented as single high voltage or multiple small stimuli. Sources of stimulation include magnetic and electrical. For magnetic tcMEP, a coil over the cortex provides the stimulation. Electrical stimulus of the motor cortex is provided by subdermal electrodes. Although occasionally associated with scalp edema and unreliable recordings, corkscrew electrodes are preferable given their low impedance and secure positioning in the scalp. Peripheral data are commonly electromyographic via CMAP. The CMAP is best monitored at sites rich in corticospinal tract innervation such as the distal limb muscles. Common recording sites are abductor pol-

licis brevis or adductor hallucis brevis with viable alternatives of long forearm flexors and extensors in the upper extremity and tibialis anterior in the lower extremity. Although there does not appear to be any monitoring advantage to increasing the number of monitored muscles, increased muscle group testing might provide a benefit in identifying positioning-related injury.

Electromyography

The clinical applications of electromyography (EMG) and its specificity for the motor system led to the introduction of spontaneous EMG (sEMG) recordings. sEMG myotomes are preselected to coordinate with operative levels, and muscle relaxants must not be utilized due to dampened or even absent activity. Continuous electrical activity to a myotome is recorded and observed and may be indicative of root irritation. When a nerve root is noted to be excessively manipulated or impinged, triggering a burst of activity, with more severe nerve manipulation and stretch of a nerve root train activity is also noted. One would generally note silence if the nerve root is cleanly severed. Distal recording sites are typically paired with an intramuscular needle or wire electrodes inserted after induction but before surgery.

Triggered EMG (tEMG) has also been used as it is postulated that a high stimulus intensity tEMG will demonstrate an intact cortex of a pedicle hole through which a screw is passed. In application, bone has high impedance requiring high threshold to stimulate the adjacent nerve. When tEMG requires high stimulation, it demonstrates the integrity of the pedicle cortex and lack of perforation. Direct stimulation of a misplaced pedicle hole with a breach, can activate the adjacent nerve root and evoke a CMAP in the appropriate myotomes at lower stimulus intensities than would be expected with an imperforate pedicle cortex. Clinical correlation is of course required, but tEMG attempts to provide data on a pathway from pedicle screw or tract to the distal site and can be used in thoracic spine operations if the rectus abdominis or intercostals musculature are monitored as the distal recording site.

Multimodality Intraoperative Monitoring

Somatosensory evoked potentials are the most common neuromonitoring modality employed, but are not always a sufficient proxy for all cord function. Failing to recognize the limitations of SSEPs can lead to devastating consequences. It must be emphasized that no single modality sufficiently monitors all spinal cord pathways. If the goal of intraoperative neuromonitoring is to detect the onset of deficits for both sensory and motor pathways, then no single modality meets the goal; however, a combination of testing methods might. Multimodality intraoperative monitoring uses all electrophysiological techniques and can provide intraoperative information about the neural structures at risk. It permits assessment of both ascending and descending pathways concurrently, providing a certain degree of redundancy because many types of intraoperative injuries will compromise both motor and sensory pathways.

Intraoperative Neurologic Complications

Significant ASD surgery requires continuous neuromonitoring, especially during placement of instrumentation and deformity correction. Immediate action is required when damage to the spinal cord or a peripheral nerve is suspected at any time during the procedure in response to changes of > 50% amplitude and > 10% latency in the SSEP/MEP signals. An algorithm may aid the primary surgeon in determining the causative factor and initiating appropriate treatment. Reassessment of neuromonitoring signal strength is performed after each step. The specific timing of each of the steps listed below is not universal; rather, timing should be determined on a case-by-case basis. Each subsequent step is initiated if the patient fails to demonstrate improvement in neurologic function after the previous sequential corrective maneuvers have been performed.

Here is a general checklist of factors to consider when SCM changes occur:

Ten-Item Checklist in Response to Losing SCM Data or Meeting Warning Criteria (SSEPs or Neurogenic MEPs)

1. Check with personnel to make certain SCM data issue is real (experience matters).
2. Be aware that an increase in blood pressure (MAP ≥ 80–90 mm Hg/systolic blood pressure > 120 mm Hg) may require a quick dose of epinephrine/norepinephrine or a dopamine drip; provide blood products if needed (hemoglobin > 9).
3. Release any traction on patient's spinal column (halo, halo-femoral, etc.).
4. Palpate the dura, checking for impingement (if spinal canal is open), such as prior osteotomies/laminectomies.
5. Reverse any corrective maneuver; also consider shortening of spinal column.
6. Confirm the absence of spinal subluxation. Consider using temporary bilateral rods during closure.
7. Consider implant malposition (screw/hook/wire) if temporally related, which might indicate dural impingement.
8. Order a wake-up test if the monitoring data have not improved or reached baseline. Also, this is a good time to take a deep breath and reflect on possible additional issues.
9. Confirm that elevated MAP is being maintained.
10. Consider apical spinal cord decompression to relieve tight neural tissue.

Increase Spinal Cord Perfusion

Immediately following identification of neuromonitoring signal changes, the hemodynamic and oxygenation status of the patient should be optimized to improve perfusion to the spinal cord. The MAP is elevated to > 80 mm Hg or 20% above baseline.[17] Hemoglobin and blood glucose levels are evaluated and corrected if required. Body temperature should be maintained at > 36.5°C to optimize neuromonitoring. These measures have been shown to increase spinal cord perfusion.[18]

Stagnara Wake-Up Test

Changes in neuromonitoring signal suggestive of persistent neurologic deficit may be cause for considering a confirmatory test. Prior to the induction of anesthesia, patients should be counseled that they will be asked to perform several commands upon awaking from anesthesia. Frequent assessment of the patient's neuromonitoring status is recommended as instrumentation is placed and corrective maneuvers performed. This enables the surgeon to most reliably pinpoint the possible inciting factor, such as a malpositioned implant or tension on the cord caused by corrective maneuvers. Thus, potentially problematic instrumentation can be removed or correction relaxed while waiting for the patient to awaken from anesthesia for the wake-up test. However, one must also understand that a time lag can occur between the application of a corrective force (e.g., distraction) and the diminution/loss of SCM signals. Thus, prudent responses to any SCM change that meets the warning criteria must be made based on the many factors involved, including the MAP, any recent correction maneuvers, and the type of data.

Release of Correction

The surgeon should consider releasing the tension on the spine when all parameters (e.g., MAP, temperature, hemoglobin level) have been reasonably addressed and there is still an absence of expected motor function with the wake-up test. After release of correction, a second wake-up test can be considered when SSEP/MEP signals indicate persistent abnormality. If an improvement in the wake-up test or in neuromonitoring is discovered after the release of surgical correction, the surgeon has the option of fusing the spine in situ or attempting a more modest correction. When no improvement in neurologic function is elicited after the release of tension, all screws and hooks should be reassessed. The stability of the spine also should be evaluated. When removal of instrumentation would compromise the stability of the spinal column, such as after vertebral body resection, the surgeon may be forced to maintain the existing instrumentation and fuse the spine under the least amount of tension. If osteotomies have been performed, the

canal should be examined for fragments of bone, Gelfoam, or bone wax, which may be contributing to cord compression.

Pedicle screw position should be critically examined in light of a monitoring change. The position of each screw can be reassessed using one measure or a combination of several. High stimulation thresholds of each fixation point, as indicated by triggered electromyography, theoretically indicate intracortical screw position secondary to increased resistance to current flow through cortical bone. Any pedicle screw with a markedly lower electromyography threshold (< 60%) in relation to the rest of the construct should be reassessed, as this may indicate a possible pedicle wall breach.[19] Screw position can also be evaluated with the use of intraoperative fluoroscopy. A pedicle screw tip past the midline of the vertebral body noted on posteroanterior radiographs is suggestive of a medial pedicle breach. In the presence of any or all of these signs, the screw may be removed to reassess the tract with direct palpation. A small laminotomy may also be performed to evaluate the integrity of the medial pedicle cortex with or without screw removal. Early removal of instrumentation may increase the possibility of neurologic improvement, provided the spine will not be significantly destabilized with removal of instrumentation.

The ability to obtain adequate postoperative imaging studies is one potential advantage of removal of instrumentation. The quality of computed tomography (CT) and MRI scans is superior when no instrumentation is present to create artifact. Even titanium constructs can produce artifact on CT or MRI scans. An MRI scan may be done in the presence of titanium instrumentation; otherwise, a CT scan can be ordered. If the instrumentation is retained and standard CT or MRI scanning is inconclusive, a CT myelogram can be performed. If an abnormality (e.g., screw malposition, hematoma) is identified, urgent return to the operating room is indicated for decompression or removal of instrumentation. If sufficient imaging can be performed and there is no identifiable site of compression, close patient observation is adequate.

Steroid Protocol

Although its use is debated, methylprednisolone is currently the only recognized pharmacologic intervention for the treatment of acute spinal cord injury (SCI).[13] The use of steroids has not been extensively studied in the intraoperative setting; however, we currently administer steroids to patients who have a continued negative wake-up test (i.e., absence of motor function) after release of tension from corrective and distractive maneuvers. The current recommended protocol is a loading intravenous bolus dose of 30 mg/kg administered over 15 minutes, followed by 5.4 mg/kg/h as a 23-hour infusion (if started within 3 hours from the time of injury).[13] The use of methylprednisolone for the management of intraoperative SCI is not well documented. Thus, the surgeon must weigh the potential benefits of improved neurologic recovery against the possible increased risk of infection. The American Association of Neurological Surgeons/Congress of Neurological Surgeons (AANS/CNS) Joint Section on Disorders of the Spine and Peripheral Nerves Guidelines Committee has indicated that methylprednisolone for either 24 or 48 hours is an option in the treatment of patients with acute SCIs that should be undertaken only with the knowledge that the evidence suggesting harmful side effects is more consistent than any suggestion of clinical benefit.

Intravenous lidocaine (2 mg/kg) for vasodilatation has been described for treatment of a postulated ischemic spinal cord after segmental vessel ligation.[20] In experimental animal models, intrathecal and intravenous vasodilators have been shown to enhance spinal cord perfusion and neuronal protection. However, we have no clinical experience with this medication and thus cannot comment specifically on its usefulness.

Postoperative Management

A patient with an intraoperative neurologic insult should be admitted to the intensive care unit postoperatively for close monitoring of hemodynamic parameters as well as for neurologic examinations. MAP must be maintained at > 80 mm Hg with the judicious use of intravenous fluid replacement, blood transfusion (if indicated), or vasopressors when necessary to maintain cord perfusion. A β-agonist (e.g., dopamine) can be used to maintain mean arterial blood pressure if fluid replacement alone is insufficient. A neurologic examination should be performed and documented every hour for the first 12 to 24 hours. This may pose a problem if the patient remains intubated and sedated. In this case, it is paramount that the patient be lightened from sedation on an hourly basis for effective assessment of neurologic function.

Delayed Postoperative Neurologic Complications

Neurologic complications in the postoperative period should be managed with the same diligence and meticulous care as described for an intraoperative SCI. Although relatively uncommon, delayed postoperative SCI may be attributed to progressive spinal cord ischemia secondary to traction or to the development of an epidural hematoma.

As with any acute SCI, adequate perfusion of the spinal cord is paramount. Blood pressure should be meticulously monitored, and MAP should be maintained at > 80 mm Hg in an effort to sustain spinal cord perfusion. Vasopressors (e.g., dopamine) may be required to attain adequate blood pressure and cord perfusion. Hemoglobin levels should also be checked to avoid excessive postoperative anemia. Patient temperature should be maintained above 36.5°C. A steroid protocol may be initiated as indicated above for the patient with continued neurologic loss.

Obtaining imaging studies before returning the patient to the operating room may aid in delineating the cause of the deficit. This will enable the surgeon to plan the proper course of action, whether that involves reexploration for localized decompression of an evolving epidural hematoma, release of correction, or removal of instrumentation to correct spinal cord ischemia secondary to excessive tensioning. Reimaging with CT or MRI scans can be omitted if obtaining these studies would result in a substantial time delay. Early decompression may improve neurologic outcome for the patient with new-onset neurologic deficit in the acute postoperative period. Conversely, if no abnormality is identified on CT or MRI scan, the patient may be observed closely with supportive treatment.

■ Chapter Summary

The surgical treatment of complex adult spinal deformity has advanced significantly in recent times with the use of pedicle screw-based instrumentation and the increasing role of complex three-column osteotomies to optimize deformity correction. The correction of large magnitude coronal and sagittal plane deformity is becoming more common. However, the technical demands involved in restoration of spinopelvic alignment and sagittal and coronal balance in large-magnitude deformities has a significant risk of neurologic complications, with potentially devastating clinical and functional sequelae. It is important that spinal surgeons use an algorithm for the safe and effective management of neurologic sequelae associated with ASD surgery so as to optimize patient management and functional outcome.

Pearls

◆ Neurologic safety during spinal deformity surgery requires preoperative preparation, intraoperative multimodality spinal cord monitoring, and postoperative diligence.
◆ A combination of SSEP, MEP, and EMG monitoring is necessary for comprehensive assessment and evaluation of neurologic function during ASD surgery.
◆ Appropriate responses to any loss of degradation of SCM data and to warning criteria should include a spectrum of responses aimed at optimizing spinal cord blood supply and minimizing any direct or indirect tension or pressure on the neural elements.
◆ To confirm the patient's neurologic integrity, one must always perform a detailed motor exam of the lower extremities at the end of the surgical procedure before the patient is extubated and leaves the operating room.

Pitfalls

◆ One must identify those patients who are at high risk of neurologic complications during ASD surgery, including those with preexisting neurologic abnormalities, an abnormal neural axis on MRI exam, or large and stiff kyphotic deformities.
◆ Not responding to or trusting the SCM personnel and data in a timely fashion can have devastating neurologic sequelae.
◆ One must be careful with those patients kept intubated/sedated following extensive ASD surgery in order not to miss a delayed neurologic complication due to the inability to obtain an adequate neurologic exam on a frequent basis.

References
Five Must-Read References

1. Dormans JP. Establishing a standard of care for neuromonitoring during spinal deformity surgery. Spine 2010;35:2180–2185
2. Malhotra NR, Shaffrey CI. Intraoperative electrophysiological monitoring in spine surgery. Spine 2010; 35:2167–2179
3. Gelalis ID, Paschos NK, Pakos EE, et al. Accuracy of pedicle screw placement: a systematic review of prospective in vivo studies comparing free hand, fluoroscopy guidance and navigation techniques. Eur Spine J 2012;21:247–255
4. Tian NF, Huang QS, Zhou P, et al. Pedicle screw insertion accuracy with different assisted methods: a systematic review and meta-analysis of comparative studies. Eur Spine J 2011;20:846–859
5. Daubs MD, Lenke LG, Cheh G, Stobbs G, Bridwell KH. Adult spinal deformity surgery: complications and outcomes in patients over age 60. Spine 2007;32: 2238–2244
6. Kim YB, Lenke LG, Kim YJ, et al. The morbidity of an anterior thoracolumbar approach: adult spinal deformity patients with greater than five-year follow-up. Spine 2009;34:822–826
7. Kim YJ, Bridwell KH, Lenke LG, Cheh G, Baldus C. Results of lumbar pedicle subtraction osteotomies for fixed sagittal imbalance: a minimum 5-year follow-up study. Spine 2007;32:2189–2197
8. Lapp MA, Bridwell KH, Lenke LG, et al. Long-term complications in adult spinal deformity patients having combined surgery a comparison of

primary to revision patients. Spine 2001;26:973–983

9. Rhee JM, Bridwell KH, Lenke LG, et al. Staged posterior surgery for severe adult spinal deformity. Spine 2003;28:2116–2121

10. Bridwell KH, Lewis SJ, Lenke LG, Baldus C, Blanke K. Pedicle subtraction osteotomy for the treatment of fixed sagittal imbalance. J Bone Joint Surg Am 2003; 85-A:454–463

11. Buchowski JM, Bridwell KH, Lenke LG, et al. Neurologic complications of lumbar pedicle subtraction osteotomy: a 10-year assessment. Spine 2007;32:2245–2252

12. Lenke LG, Fehlings MG, Shaffrey CI, et al. Prospective, multicenter assessment of acute neurologic complications following complex adult spinal deformity surgery: the Scoli-Risk-1 trial. Spine 2014 submitted

13. Winter RB. Neurologic safety in spinal deformity surgery. Spine 1997;22:1527–1533

14. Owen JH. The application of intraoperative monitoring during surgery for spinal deformity. Spine 1999; 24:2649–2662

15. Vauzelle C, Stagnara P, Jouvinroux P. Functional monitoring of spinal cord activity during spinal surgery. Clin Orthop Relat Res 1973;93:173–178

16. Lesser RP, Raudzens P, Lüders H, et al. Postoperative neurological deficits may occur despite unchanged intraoperative somatosensory evoked potentials. Ann Neurol 1986;19:22–25

17. Naslund TC, Hollier LH, Money SR, Facundus EC, Skenderis BS II. Protecting the ischemic spinal cord during aortic clamping. The influence of anesthetics and hypothermia. Ann Surg 1992;215:409–415, discussion 415–416

18. Raynor BL, Lenke LG, Kim Y, et al. Can triggered electromyograph thresholds predict safe thoracic pedicle screw placement? Spine 2002;27:2030–2035

19. Bracken MB, Shepard MJ, Holford TR, et al. Administration of methylprednisolone for 24 or 48 hours or tirilazad mesylate for 48 hours in the treatment of acute spinal cord injury. Results of the Third National Acute Spinal Cord Injury Randomized Controlled Trial. National Acute Spinal Cord Injury Study. JAMA 1997;277:1597–1604

20. Klemme WR, Burkhalter W, Polly DW Jr, Dahl LF, Davis DA. Reversible ischemic myelopathy during scoliosis surgery: a possible role for intravenous lidocaine. J Pediatr Orthop 1999;19:763–765

7

Postoperative Coronal Decompensation in Adult Deformity

Yong Qiu

■ General Introduction of Adult Scoliosis

Adult scoliosis is defined as an abnormal deformity in an adult, with Cobb angle greater than 10 degrees in the coronal plane, with or without sagittal imbalance or abnormal pelvic orientation.[1] In the elderly population, a variety of prevalence rates have been reported as a result of differences in definitions of scoliosis, sample size, ethnicity, and screening tools. In a study of volunteers who were over 60 years of age, Schwab et al[2] found that 68% of the subjects met the definition of scoliosis. As reported by Xu et al,[3] the prevalence of scoliosis was 13.3% in a cohort of 2395 adults older than 40 years of age.

Adult scoliosis may stem from progression of scoliosis during childhood or adolescence (**Fig. 7.1**), or may be newly developed in adulthood through degenerative changes (**Fig. 7.2**). The former condition is referred to adult idiopathic scoliosis, whereas the latter is termed degenerative scoliosis or de novo scoliosis. In contrast to adolescents, adults with scoliosis characteristically present with back pain, radiculopathy, and neurogenic claudication. Cosmesis is a concern of some young adult scoliosis patients. They often complain of waist asymmetry and ribs abutting the pelvis, as a result of imbalance in the coronal plane or the sagittal plane.

For adult scoliosis, nonoperative care is usually the first-line treatment option. Nevertheless, surgery may be inevitable when nonoperative measures fail. The primary indications for surgery of adult scoliosis are (1) progressive deformity, (2) poor spinal balance causing functional difficulties, (3) large deformity threatening cardiopulmonary compromise, (4) neurologic manifestations, (5) persistent pain that fails to respond to nonoperative treatment, and (6) unacceptable cosmetic appearance.[1,4–6] Bess et al,[7] in a multicenter review of 290 patients with adult scoliosis, reported that operative treatment for older patients was primarily driven by pain and disability, independent of radiographic measurements, and, for younger patients, by increased coronal plane deformity. Although operative management of adult scoliosis is a growing challenge, a variety of surgical options has been employed, include posterior, anterior, or combined approaches. Silva and Lenke[6] proposed six distinct levels of surgical options for adult degenerative scoliosis: I, decompression alone; II, decompression and limited instrumented posterior spinal fusion; III, decompression and lumbar curve instrumented fusion; IV, decompression with anterior and posterior spinal instrumented fusion; V, thoracic instrumentation and fusion extension; and VI, inclusion of osteotomies for specific deformities.

Fusion levels should start proximally at a stable vertebra, typically above T6 or below

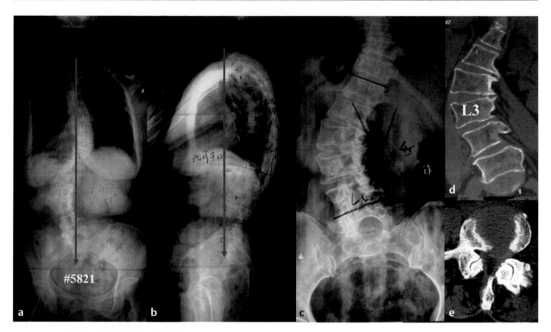

Fig. 7.1a–e (a,b) A 57-year-old woman with a history of adolescent idiopathic scoliosis. **(c–e)** Both coronal and global sagittal balance was well maintained, and the L2/3 disk height was much better preserved on the convex side than on the concave side.

T10, and end distally at a neutral and stable vertebra. The proximal level never starts at the thoracic kyphosis apex, avoiding proximal junctional kyphosis, whereas the distal level never ends at a level with rotatory subluxation. The decision of whether to include L5 or the sacrum in the fusion is controversial.[8,9] Fusion distally to L5 offers the theoretical benefits of preserved lumbosacral motion, shorter surgical time, and a decreased likelihood of pseudarthrosis; on the other hand, it carries the potential for accelerated symptomatic advanced degeneration at the L5/S1 disk, which in turn ultimately results in axial discomfort, radiculopathy, and loss of lumbosacral lordosis. In contrast to L5, fusions extended to the sacrum achieve a higher stability of fixation as well as a better correction of sagittal imbalance, but this procedure also runs the risk of an increasing chance of pseudarthrosis, a greater frequency of major complications, and a higher rate of instrumentation failure.[8,9] A recent study also found fusion to the sacrum to be one of the risk factors of proximal junctional kyphosis.[10] Noncontroversial indications for fusion to the sa-

crum include the following[6]: (1) an oblique take-off of L5 on the sacrum, (2) a lumbosacral fractional curve > 15 degrees, (3) advanced degeneration of the L5/S1 disk or the L5/S1 facet joints, (4) L5/S1 spondylolisthesis, and (5) prior history of decompression at this segment. When fusion to the sacrum cannot be avoided, it is important to perform an interbody fusion between L5 and S1 to decrease the risk of a nonunion.

■ Differentiating Between Degenerative and Idiopathic Scoliosis

An essential premise of the treatment of spinal deformity in particular is understanding its etiology. Aebi[1] developed in 2005 a classification for adult scoliosis based on the etiology: type 1, de novo scoliosis; type 2, progressive idiopathic scoliosis; type 3a, secondary degenerative scoliosis, due to a preexisting condition, either intrinsic (adjacent curve) or extrinsic

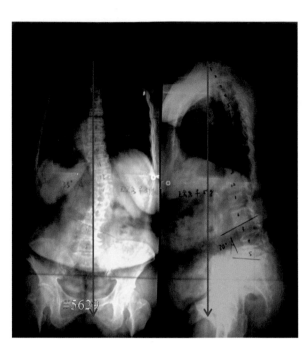

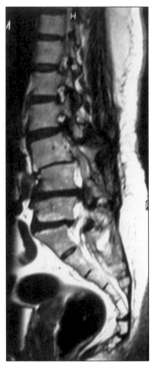

a

b

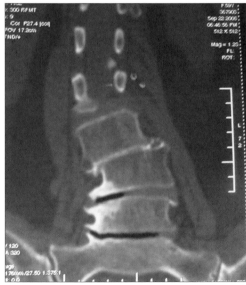

c

d

Fig. 7.2a–d Adult degenerative scoliosis in a 65-year-old woman. **(a)** Standing X-ray films showed a right-sided lumbar curve, rotatory subluxation at L3/4, and regional kyphosis from L3 to L5 as well as sagittal imbalance. **(b)** Magnetic resonance imaging of advanced disk degeneration showed dark disks with narrowed disk height. **(c,d)** Computed tomography scans demonstrated the vacuum phenomenon as well as canal stenosis in the lower lumbar region.

(lower limb length discrepancy) to the spine; and type 3b, scoliosis secondary to metabolic bone disease. However, it is difficult to differentiate the clinical etiology in elderly patients who are unable to provide either a medical history or information about their spinal deformity. As there is a paucity of information in the literature, this chapter describes several experience-based radiographic criteria that may help to differentiate between de novo and idiopathic scoliosis.

Apical Disk Height

In de novo scoliosis, asymmetrical disk degeneration has been regarded as the initiating factor that contributes to the occurrence of degenerative scoliosis. Asymmetric degeneration in the apical disks leads to asymmetric disk collapse, inducing a curvature by pivoting on the apical facet joint at the concave side, which in turn exacerbates more degeneration of the disks on the concave side than on the convex side and then start the vicious circle. Bao et al[11] also found that regional lumbar disk degeneration correlated with the coronal Cobb angle, confirming that asymmetric disk degeneration contributed to the development of de novo scoliosis. We observed that the convex disk height was significantly less in de novo scoliosis (**Fig. 7.2**) than in idiopathic scoliosis (**Fig. 7.1**).

Curve Pattern

The majority of degenerative scoliosis affects the lumbar or thoracolumbar spine, and their curve patterns may be different from that of idiopathic scoliosis. Because the original pathogenesis of de novo scoliosis is the degeneration of disk and facet joints, the apex of the lumbar curve is often located at the intervertebral space. The most common apex of de novo scoliosis is the intervertebral space of L2/3 or L3/4, often with a shorter curve span. In addition, the levels involved in the degenerative curve are generally three to four levels, whereas four

to six levels are more common in idiopathic curves.

Regularity of Apical Vertebra

In addition to curve patterns, the apical vertebra in de novo scoliosis is often irregularly wedged. Osteophytes, end-plate abruption, and osteoporotic minor fracture are commonly seen in degenerative vertebrae, so the shape of vertebra may not be regularly trapezoid. In contrast, wedging of apical vertebra, if any, is usually regular in idiopathic lumbar scoliosis.

Compensatory Curve Above the Main Curve

Regular compensatory curves proximal to the main curve in idiopathic scoliosis may develop during adolescence, and serve as a way to rebalance the distal thoracolumbar/lumbar curve in the coronal plane (**Fig. 7.1**). That explains why global coronal imbalance is less frequent in adolescent idiopathic scoliosis cases with double curve patterns, owing to the compensatory curve and its compensatory ability from the diskal, pelvic, and certainly spinal muscular structure as well. This balancing pattern may continue into adulthood and last for a long time. This feature of compensatory curves could serve as an important radiographic sign to differentiate these two entities.

Patients with de novo scoliosis often present early with coronal or sagittal imbalance due to the less effective compensative curves above the imbalance. In contrast with sagittal imbalance, there is paucity of information in the literature on the incidence of coronal imbalance in de novo scoliosis. Based on our study,[11] about one third of patients with de novo scoliosis may present with coronal imbalance due to a lack of compensatory curves. Similar to the functional scoliosis seen in young individuals with disk herniation or other lower back diseases, trunk shifting is not uncommon in de novo scoliosis with stenosis because of the pain-alleviating mechanism. This trunk shifting or coronal imbalance with spinal curve may become structural with time.

Correlation Between the Cobb Angle and Imbalance

The discrepancy between the Cobb angle and imbalance in de novo scoliosis is an interesting finding. Degenerative curves always are shorter than the idiopathic curves and have a smaller Cobb angle. As mentioned earlier, coronal imbalance is an important feature of de novo scoliosis, whatever the Cobb angle, whereas significant imbalance is mostly witnessed in adult idiopathic scoliosis with severe curves. Therefore, a small Cobb angle with obvious coronal imbalance indicates that the curve might be degenerative (**Fig. 7.2**).

Correction Ability of Rotatory Subluxation

Vertebral rotatory subluxation (VRS) is a triaxial deformity, predominantly at the L3/L4 level, with female predominance. Although it is more likely to occur in patients with de novo scoliosis at the early stage of the deformity, it could also occur during the late course of adult idiopathic scoliosis. At our center, we found that the correct ability of VRS under traction or on side-bending films could be used to differentiate de novo scoliosis and idiopathic scoliosis. In the former, reduction of VRS under traction or on side bending may not be achieved because of the rigidity from vertebral degeneration at the subluxation level, including disk collapse, osteophytes, and spontaneous vertebral or facet fusion. In contrast, in idiopathic scoliosis, VRS could be partially reduced under traction or on side bending.

Discrepancy Between the Cobb Angle and Rotatory Subluxation

At our center we noted that VRS was more like to occur when the Cobb angle increased in cases of idiopathic scoliosis. However, in de novo scoliosis, VRS may occur at its early stage, and its onset and severity may not necessarily be correlated with the Cobb angle. In other words, VRS in de novo scoliosis may develop even in cases with a small curve.

The Origin of Stenosis

According to the definition of de novo scoliosis, its primary cause is the degeneration of spine, including disks, the muscle–ligaments complex, and the facet joint. Lumbar stenosis is more commonly seen in primary degenerative scoliosis than in adult idiopathic curves. Therefore, radicular leg pain and claudication should be more common in de novo scoliosis, even with small curves. This is in accordance with our clinical observation that mechanical back pain is the most common complaint in many adult idiopathic scoliosis patients due to deformity-induced paraspinal muscle fatigue, whereas neurogenic back pain in combination with leg pain is the most common complaint in de novo scoliosis patients (**Fig. 7.2**).

Lumbar Lordosis

In addition to different curve presentations in the coronal plane, sagittal alignment may also be different between de novo and idiopathic scoliosis, especially in the early stages. Lumbar lordosis may remain normal in idiopathic scoliosis because disk height may be maintained for a long time. In de novo scoliosis, however, lumbar lordosis may not be preserved because of early disk collapse. Bao et al[11] also demonstrated that de novo scoliosis patients with severe disk degeneration have lumbar hypolordosis or kyphosis (**Fig. 7.2**). Moreover, osteoporotic fracture is more frequently observed in de novo scoliosis, particularly in female patients, greatly contributing to lumbar kyphosis, whereas in idiopathic scoliosis, the degenerative pathologies are not the primary cause, and osteoporotic fracture may be less common.

Contribution of Disk Degeneration to Spinal Imbalance and Curve Severity

Spine imbalance in the sagittal or coronal plane has an important impact on the health status and treatment options in patients with de novo scoliosis. Sagittal imbalance is closely correlated with poor health-related quality of life (HRQOL). Importantly, it has been well documented that coronal imbalance is also one of the main causes of unsatisfactory appearance, impaired function, and back pain.[12] Because the established consensus in terms of the origin of de novo scoliosis is that it is triggered by asymmetrical disk degeneration, our team conducted a study specifically focused on the correlation between disk degeneration and spinal imbalance.[11]

We quantified disk degeneration using the Pfirrmann classification, which describes five grades of disk degeneration on magnetic resonance imaging.[13] Each grade of disk was scored with a specific number to enable doing calculations; for example, grade I was given a score of 5, whereas grade V was given a score of 1. Thus, higher scores represented healthier disk conditions.

The results of our study revealed that disk degeneration at the lower end vertebra (EV) was strongly correlated with sagittal imbalance (**Fig. 7.2**). We found that the grade of the lower EV disk reached a mean degeneration score of 2.32, being the second most severely degenerated disk after the apical disk. There may be three stages of disk degeneration, correlated with stability and motion: dysfunction, instability, and stabilization. With moderate disk degeneration, the disk might become unstable. Also, there might be a tendency for instability to lie in moderately degenerated disks with well-preserved disk height, whereas mobility may decrease and restabilize in the collapsed disks. This finding supported our assumption that lower EV disk degeneration was more responsible for the sagittal imbalance because its stability was jeopardized. However, we failed to find significant correlation between coronal imbalance and disk degeneration. Certainly, degeneration of the posterior elements, including the facet joints and the paraspinal muscle, is another accepted factor accounting for de novo scoliosis; therefore, it is assumed that unstable posterior elements instead of disk degeneration may be the important cause of coronal imbalance in lumbar degenerative scoliosis. The degenerative facet joints with osteoarthritis may be the primary cause, or may be secondary to the loss of disk height, leading to vertebral instability and increased segmental axial mobility, which may contribute to coronal imbalance. Asymmetric atrophy of paraspinal muscles is another possible factor influencing coronal balance. The degree of instability varies in each individual, based on the slip in the sagittal plane, translational dislocations in the coronal plane, and three-dimensional rotational subluxation.

Correlation between the Cobb angle and apical disk degeneration was also noted. The more degeneration the apical disk presented, the larger is the Cobb angle. Such a close relationship between degeneration of the apical disk and the Cobb angle can be explained by the pathology of degenerative scoliosis: asymmetric degeneration in the apical disk will lead to asymmetric disk collapse, inducing the spine to bend the apical facet joints, which in turn exacerbates the degeneration of the concave side. In addition, we also found that regional lumbar disk degeneration grade is correlated with sagittal malalignment, including an anteverted C7PL and lumbar kyphosis (**Fig. 7.2**). Decreases in lumbar lordosis in patients with disk degeneration, as evidenced in our study, explain why de novo scoliosis patients with severely degenerated disks had lumbar hypolordosis or kyphosis.

Coronal Balance of Adult Deformity

Coronal Balance Assessment

The concept of balance of the spine has been extensively described by the *Scoliosis Research Society* (SRS). The concept implies that, in both the coronal and sagittal planes, the head is positioned correctly over the sacrum and pelvis, in both a translational and an angular sense. From the frontal view of the trunk, balance implies horizontal shoulders and the trunk evenly distributed about the vertical line passing through the center sacral vertical line (CSVL). Spinal balance in the coronal plane can be determined as the displacement of the most cephalad vertebra from the CSVL in both a distance (frontal plane offset) and an angle (offset angle). In practice, the defined cephalad vertebra usually is C7 or T1 (**Fig. 7.3**). Compensation in the coronal plane is usually referred to as the translation of the midpoint of C7 in relation to CSVL (measured in the same manner as coronal balance [CB]). It primarily describes the position of the head over the pelvis. Decompensation occurs when this alignment strays from the midline by more than a threshold value specified by the investigators, usually reported as 2 cm.

The word *balance* implies a static alignment in the standing (or unsupported seated) position, whereas *compensation* and *decompensation* refer to the result of dynamic alignment. In detail, *compensation* signifies the active process of becoming balanced, whereas *decompensation* indicates a failure to achieve balance, especially after an intervention such as surgery.

Relationship Between Coronal Balance and Quality of Life

In patients with adult scoliosis, the impact of sagittal balance on clinical health status has

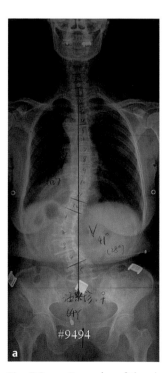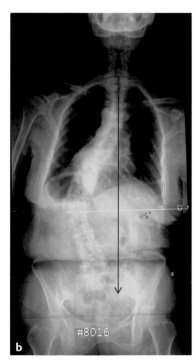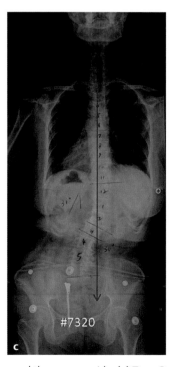

Fig. 7.3a–c Examples of the classification of the coronal balance pattern in adult scoliosis. **(a)** Type A in a 64-year-old woman without obvious truncal asymmetry. **(b)** Type B in a 63-year-old woman with the trunk shifting toward the concave side. **(c)** Type C in a 61-year-old woman with the trunk shifting toward the convex side.

been extensively discussed, whereas the impact of coronal balance on functional outcomes is less clear. In contrast to patients with idiopathic scoliosis, patients with degenerative lumbar scoliosis have an increased likelihood of imbalance in the coronal plane. Because of asymmetrical degenerative changes and vertebral wedging in the apical region, coronal imbalance is frequently observed. According to the study by Daubs et al,[14] 13 of 85 (15%) adult scoliosis patients with preoperative coronal imbalance had worsening coronal balance of more than 1 cm after surgery. This finding suggests that the incidence of postoperative imbalance in the coronal plane is underestimated.

It has been found that coronal imbalance correlates with significant clinical manifestations such as pelvic obliquity, sitting or standing imbalance, as well as severe cosmetic truncal deformity. Moreover, coronal imbalance is one of the main underlying causes of the progression of deformity, back pain, and functional compromise. Axial pain usually derives from the convexity of the curve, and leads to further deterioration of coronal imbalance. Radicular pain and neurogenic claudication mainly originate from the compression on the concavity of the curve, or from dynamic overstretching on the convex side.[1] Deterioration of these symptoms runs in parallel with the increase in coronal imbalance to some extent. To address these problems, it is important to correct the preoperative coronal imbalance.

To help elucidate the factors that are most crucial for improved outcomes, several studies have attempted to correlate radiographic findings with clinical symptoms in adult scoliosis. Glassman et al[15] reported that significant coronal imbalance was associated with pain and dysfunction in unoperated patients, and coronal imbalance was not as critical a parameter as sagittal imbalance in prediction of symptoms. However, Daubs et al[14] showed that sagittal balance is the strongest predictor of improved functional outcomes in adult scoliosis patients. They found that restoring sagittal balance in patients with combined coronal and sagittal imbalance seems to be the key to improving the functional outcomes. In terms of patients with coronal imbalance alone, improvement in

coronal balance was a significant predictor of improved surgical outcomes.[14]

In some studies, coronal imbalance has also been reported to lead to decreased HRQOL and increased risk of implant failure in adult scoliosis patients.[15-17] In the study by Glassman et al,[15] significant coronal imbalance of greater than 4 cm was associated with more pain and dysfunction for unoperated patients but not for operated patients. Ploumis et al[16] reported that patients with coronal imbalance of greater than 50 mm showed worse physical function scores. Cho et al[17] demonstrated that preoperative coronal imbalance led to more implant failures, requiring removal of the implant. Therefore, improved postoperative coronal balance should be the goal in order to improve the HRQOL as well as to reduce the need for revision surgery. At our center, postoperative coronal imbalance was one of the factors that contributed to implant failure.

Decompensation in the Coronal Plane

As mentioned above, decompensation in the coronal plane implies dynamic malalignment of the spine, commonly measured as CB (translation of the center of C7 in relation to CSVL) beyond a specified threshold value. In adolescent idiopathic scoliosis patients, decompensation was usually defined as coronal imbalance of more than 2 cm (measured in the same manner as CB). In adult scoliosis patients, the threshold value of decompensation in the coronal plane varied among studies. Glassman et al[15] reported the association between coronal imbalance of greater than 4 cm and deterioration in clinical symptoms in nonoperated patients. Daubs et al[14] and Ploumis et al[16] defined coronal imbalance as C7PL > 4 cm and > 5 cm lateral to CSVL, respectively. In a recent study, with emphasis on coronal imbalance in adult spinal deformity patients treated with long fusions, Ploumis et al[18] also employed a criterion of 4 cm.

In a study by the SRS that classified adult scoliosis according to the King/Moe and Lenke classifications, coronal imbalance was considered to be one of the global balance modifiers.[19]

Imbalance was considered to be present if the C7PL was located > 3 cm to the right or left of the CSVL. We recently surveyed a consecutive series of degenerative lumbar scoliosis patients to evaluate coronal balance, with the balance threshold set at 3 cm. We found a high prevalence of preoperative coronal imbalance in adults with degenerative lumbar scoliosis. In these patients, imbalance occurred either on the concave side, namely C7 deviating toward the concave side of the main curve with reference to CSVL (**Fig. 7.3b**), or on the convex side, with C7 deviating toward the convex side (**Fig. 7.3c**).

Postoperative Coronal Decompensation

Postoperative coronal decompensation is a major complication in adult scoliosis.[14,18] In addition to the Daubs et al[14] finding reported above (see section Relationship Between Coronal Balance and Quality of Life), Ploumis et al,[18] in a cohort of 54 adult patients treated with long fusions, found postoperative coronal decompensation in seven patients with preoperative coronal imbalance and in four without, at six weeks postoperatively. At a minimum 2-year follow-up, four more patients without initial imbalance were observed with coronal decompensation. The authors reported that postoperative coronal decompensation was found in an increased number of adult spine deformity patients.[18] But so far, the underlying factors that predict postoperative coronal decompensation remain unclear.

In theory, decreased compensation of the segments above and below the fusion predisposes the patient to postoperative coronal decompensation. Multiple deformity- and surgery-related factors are probably associated with the occurrence of postoperative coronal decompensation.

Deformity-Related Factors

We found that the preoperative coronal imbalance pattern plays an important role in the occurrence of postoperative coronal decompensation. A curve with imbalance to the convex side predisposes to further decompensation, particularly when osteotomies of the posterior elements, such as Smith-Petersen osteotomy (SPO), or through three columns, such as pedicle subtraction osteotomy (PSO), are undertaken.[6,20] For cases with imbalance to the convex side, compression maneuvers on the convex side at the level(s) of the osteotomy, which are performed to close the osteotomy gap, may lead to further inclination of the trunk toward the convex side. As in congenital thoracolumbar kyphoscoliosis, we also noticed that patients with preoperative convex imbalance had a higher rate of postoperative coronal decompensation after three-column osteotomies.

At the same time, decreased compensation above and below the instrumentation also play an important role in the development of postoperative coronal decompensation, because the compensation potential of the unfused segments comes mainly from the disks and paravertebral musculature. Hence, the more degenerative changes the adjacent vertebrae cephalad or caudal to the fusion levels manifest, the worse the potential ability for these unfused segments to compensate, resulting in an increasing likelihood of postoperative coronal decompensation.

Surgery-Related Factors

Among the surgery-related factors that have impact on the occurrence of postoperative coronal decompensation, the lower instrumented vertebra (LIV) selection is of upmost importance. Ending LIV at a vertebra that cannot become horizontal during surgery carries the potential risk of postoperative decompensation. If there is a residual obliquity of LIV in the coronal plane, an inclination of the trunk is bound to occur, because the disk below LIV provides limited range of motion. As mentioned previously, we found that the disks of the lower lumbar region showed significant degenerative changes. The physiological function of these disks is correspondingly compromised. Apparently, fusion distally stopping at a vertebra that cannot become horizontal places the coronal balance pattern at risk of decompensation after surgery.

In addition, proper determination of the upper instrumented vertebra (UIV) can diminish the incidence of coronal decompensation. A location of UIV below the end vertebra of the main curve can result in inclination of the fusion with reference to the CSVL. If fusion extends into the thoracic region, however, a much more cephalad location of the UIV than the end vertebra also carries the risk of decompensation, because it lowers the number of thoracic vertebrae with compensation potential. Moreover, inclination of UIV to the convex side of the main curve probably impedes balance in the coronal plane through the adverse impact on the auto-compensation mechanism.

An inappropriate osteotomy algorithm may contribute to postoperative coronal decompensation as well. Three-column osteotomies usually begin at the apex and from the convex side.[20] This is effective in the correction of cases with preoperative coronal imbalance to the concave side. For a case with preexistent imbalance to the convex side, however, such a maneuver might aggravate the imbalance because of the compression forces at the osteotomized site from the convex side.

In practice, surgeons perform sagittal balance restoration more than in the coronal plane, and the balance pattern and the compensation potential in the coronal plane are sometimes ignored. Such an attitude toward coronal plane balance is evidently an underlying risk factor for postoperative coronal decompensation. Multiple studies have demonstrated that coronal imbalance accompanied by sagittal imbalance is a more common clinical scenario.[14,16,19] Therefore, adequate attention needs to be paid not only to the sagittal plane but also to the coronal plane. In patients complaining of sagittal imbalance, Bridwell[20] classified the coexistent coronal imbalance with into type A and type B. In type A, the patient's shoulders and pelvis are tilted in opposite directions; the shoulder is elevated at the side where the pelvis is lower. Conversely, with type B, both the shoulders and the pelvis tilt in the same direction. An asymmetrical PSO is often useful in correcting type A biplanar deformities.[21] The more radical techniques such as vertebral column resection (VCR) are sometimes useful for the rare type B deformities.[20]

Prevention of Postoperative Coronal Decompensation

A Novel Classification of Coronal Balance Pattern

A discrepancy exists between sagittal imbalance, which is well accounted for in the traditional treatment algorithm, and imbalance in the coronal plane, which the algorithm ignores. Furthermore, postoperative coronal decompensation is an important complication that affects surgical outcome and increases the revision rate. To address this problem, we have established a novel classification regarding coronal balance patterns for adult scoliosis.

This classification is based on CB, which is measured as the distance of the midpoint of C7 relative to the CSVL on standing posteroanterior X-ray films (**Fig. 7.3**). Vertebral alignment in the coronal plane is considered to be balanced if CB is less than 3 cm at either side; otherwise, it is considered to be imbalanced. Patients with a balanced coronal pattern are categorized as type A (**Fig. 7.3a**). Patients with an imbalanced coronal pattern (CB more than 3 cm) are categorized as type B if the imbalance is on the concave side of the main curve (**Fig. 7.3b**) and type C if the imbalance is on the convex side of the main curve (**Fig. 7.3c**).

Osteotomy Options Based on This Classification

For a coronal pattern of type A or type B, the three-column osteotomy, if necessary, should be performed right at the apex from the convex side, so as to restore lumbar lordosis and to reestablish coronal balance when the compression forces are applied to close the osteotomy gap. This osteotomy option is very effective in correcting patients with a type B coronal pattern. But in type C patients with preoperative coronal imbalance on the convex side, this osteotomy option might be inappropriate due to the compression forces at the apex. Although it is rare, intraoperative dislocation after three-column osteotomy can occur as a severe complication, due to compulsively rectifying the imbalanced trunk, which is accompanied by a relatively rigid lumbosacral hemicurve.

To restore a balanced spine with the trunk centrally over the pelvis, a novel osteotomy strategy has been suggested for cases with type C (**Fig. 7.4**). First, a three-column osteotomy needs to be performed at a more distal level, usually at the L4 vertebra or the L4/5 disk from the concave side of the main curve to restore the balance of the trunk over the pelvis. Second, the apical region is then corrected. In cases with kyphosis, an additional three-column osteotomy can be done at the apex. The optimal strategy of osteotomy for type C begins from the concave side, and converts the previous imbalance pattern into a type A pattern.

In addition, an asymmetrical PSO might be an alternate option for patients with a type C pattern. Toyone et al[21] described the technique of asymmetrical PSO through which a coronal correction was well achieved upon closure of the osteotomy wedge on the convex side.

■ Revision Surgery for Instrumentation Failure Due to Postoperative Coronal Imbalance

Long spinal instrumentation is often indicated in adult spinal deformity, which immobilizes a long span of spinal segments, leading to increased motion of the adjacent segments and the potential for degenerative pathology. Because the lumbosacral junction presents high mechanical demand, a high rate of complications has been well documented for long fusions to the sacrum. One of the implant-related complications is rod fracture, which is associated with the use of iliac screws or small-diameter rods, operating at inappropriate fusion levels, resulting in postoperative coronal imbalance, and failing to address sagittal imbalance.

Postoperative coronal imbalance often requires additional revision surgery. In our practice, the incidence of rod breakage is 15% in adult spinal deformity patients (9/59) with a minimum of 2-year follow-up, particularly in patients with postoperative residual kyphosis. We speculate that rod fracture may partly result from overloaded mechanical forces imposed on instrumentation in cases with postoperative coronal imbalance (**Fig. 7.5**).

The use of iliac screws might increase the risk of implant failure because of the increased stiffness of the lumbosacral constructs. The excessive stress of rod contouring is necessary to connect iliac screws and S1 pedicle screws, but it can lead to rod fracture.[22] In particular, we found that, in patients with postoperative coronal decompensation, the location of the rod fracture is often close to the level of the iliac crest or the osteotomy level (**Fig. 7.6**).

Postoperative coronal imbalance that is complicated by a symptomatic rod fracture is a definitive indication for revision surgery. Several modalities have been employed to fix the fractured rod. Traditionally, the entire incision is reopened and the fractured rod is replaced with a new one. Alternatively, revision with a combination of in-line rod connectors and crosslinks can restore the stiffness of the original construct without the need to replace the entire construct. To reinforce the local construction of the fractured rod and decrease the risk of complications, we use satellite rods (**Fig. 7.6**). This local direct-repair strategy requires the reopening of only the area surrounding the fractured rod rather than the entire opening along the instrumentation. More importantly, satellite rods can enable the restoration of coronal balance through local compression at the convex side or distraction at the concave side. Recently, we started using the satellite rods in the index surgery at the osteotomy level or when the instrumentation bridges the lumbosacral junction.

■ Chapter Summary

Adult scoliosis may stem from the progression of scoliosis in children or adolescents (idiopathic type), or may newly develop in adulthood through degenerative changes (degenerative

(*text continues on page 93*)

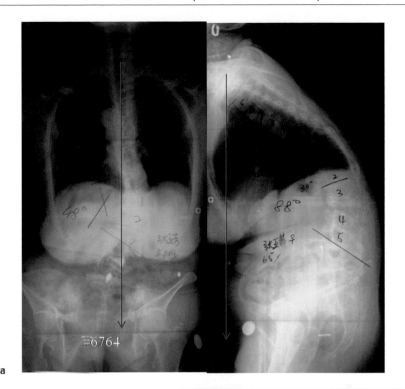

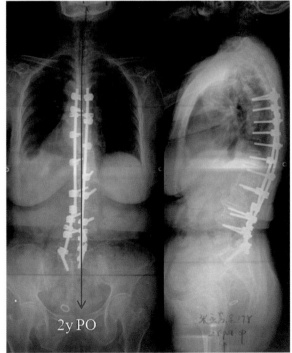

Fig. 7.4a,b (a) A 65-year-old woman with degenerative scoliosis and a type C coronal balance pattern. Lumbar kyphosis and severe sagittal imbalance was noted. As per the surgical algorithm, a long fusion from T6 to S1 was started with osteotomy at L4/5 to balance the spine in the coronal plane followed by a pedicle subtraction osteotomy (PSO) at L1. **(b)** At 2-year follow-up, the spinal balance was well maintained.

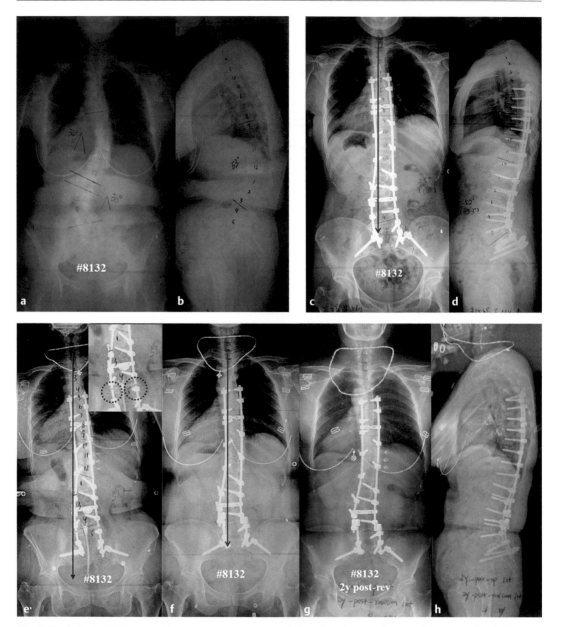

Fig. 7.5a–h (a,b) A 56-year-old woman with degenerative lumbar kyphoscoliosis complicated by lumbar stenosis. Posterior spinal fusion from T5 to pelvis was done together with L4-L5 decompression. **(c,d)** Postoperative coronal imbalance was noted. **(e)** Both rods were fractured at 8 months' follow-up. **(f)** Revision surgery with a domino connector was performed to restore coronal balance, which was well maintained at **(g,h)** 2 years, follow-up.

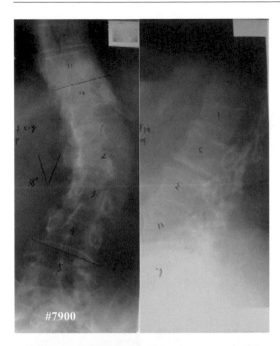

Fig. 7.6a–e **(a,b)** A 64-year-old woman with degenerative lumbar scoliosis was treated with Luque instrumentation 9 years ago in another hospital. Posterior instrumentation from T5 to S1 with an L1 PSO was performed in the revision surgery. **(c)** However, immediate postoperative coronal imbalance toward the convex side was noted. (*continued on page 92*)

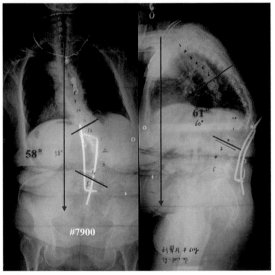

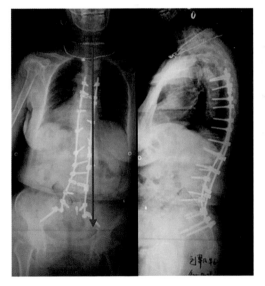

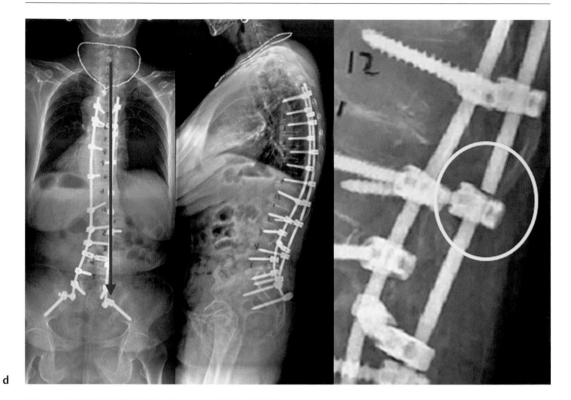

d

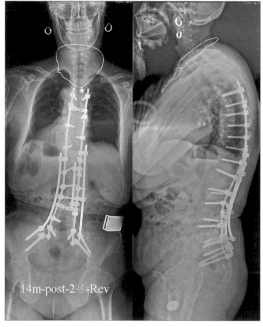

14m-post-2nd-Rev

e

Fig. 7.6a–e (*continued*) **(d)** Two years later, the rod fractured at the right side of L2. **(e)** A second revision surgery was performed with satellite rods. Both coronal and sagittal balance was restored at 6 months' follow-up.

type). Surgical interventions are mainly indicated for patients complaining of pain and disability. In our experience, several factors differentiate between degenerative and idiopathic scoliosis. In degenerative scoliosis, disk degeneration contributes to the occurrence of spinal imbalance. Disk degeneration at the lower end vertebra strongly correlates with sagittal imbalance, whereas that at the apex correlates with curve magnitude. In degenerative lumbar scoliosis, imbalance in the coronal plane is frequently observed and usually associated with deterioration of symptoms such as back pain and radiculopathy. A recent survey found a high rate of preoperative coronal imbalance in degenerative lumbar scoliosis, on either the concave or the convex side. Corrective surgery might result in coronal decompensation in adult scoliosis patients, leading to trunk shifting and possibly implant failure. Deformity- and surgery-related factors might lead to this complication.

A novel classification system has been devised for the coronal balance pattern in adult scoliosis: type A, balanced; type B, imbalanced on the concave side; and type C, imbalanced on the convex side. For a preoperative coronal pattern of type A or B, the three-column osteotomy should be performed right at the apex from the convex side. For type C, the optimal strategy of osteotomy begins from the concave side of the main curve, at a more distal level, usually at the L4 vertebra or L4/5 disk, followed by correction of the apical region. For instrumentation failure due to postoperative coronal decompensation, revision surgery focuses on reinforcing the local construction, using in-line rod connectors, cross-links, or satellite rods.

Pearls

- Consult the classification system that has been devised for preoperative coronal balance pattern in adult scoliosis.
- Identify the factors that differentiate degenerative and idiopathic adult scoliosis.
- Keep in mind that disk degeneration may contribute to spinal imbalance and curve severity.
- Evaluate the risk factors of postoperative coronal decompensation.
- Be aware of revision options for instrumentation failure due to postoperative coronal imbalance.

Pitfalls

- Postoperative coronal decompensation can occur after osteotomy at the apex.
- Postoperative coronal decompensation may result in instrumentation failure and loss of correction.

References
Five Must-Read References

1. Aebi M. The adult scoliosis. Eur Spine J 2005;14: 925–948
2. Schwab F, Dubey A, Gamez L, et al. Adult scoliosis: prevalence, SF-36, and nutritional parameters in an elderly volunteer population. Spine 2005;30:1082–1085
3. Xu L, Sun X, Huang S, et al. Degenerative lumbar scoliosis in Chinese Han population: prevalence and relationship to age, gender, bone mineral density, and body mass index. Eur Spine J 2013;22:1326–1331
4. Glassman SD, Schwab FJ, Bridwell KH, Ondra SL, Berven S, Lenke LG. The selection of operative versus nonoperative treatment in patients with adult scoliosis. Spine 2007;32:93–97
5. Smith JS, Shaffrey CI, Berven S, et al; Spinal Deformity Study Group. Operative versus nonoperative treatment of leg pain in adults with scoliosis: a retrospective review of a prospective multicenter database with two-year follow-up. Spine 2009;34:1693–1698
6. Silva FE, Lenke LG. Adult degenerative scoliosis: evaluation and management. Neurosurg Focus 2010; 28:E1
7. Bess S, Boachie-Adjei O, Burton D, et al; International Spine Study Group. Pain and disability determine treatment modality for older patients with adult scoliosis, while deformity guides treatment for younger patients. Spine 2009;34:2186–2190
8. Bridwell KH, Edwards CC II, Lenke LG. The pros and cons to saving the L5-S1 motion segment in a long scoliosis fusion construct. Spine 2003;28(20, Suppl): S234–S242
9. Polly DW Jr, Hamill CL, Bridwell KH. Debate: to fuse or not to fuse to the sacrum, the fate of the L5-S1 disc. Spine 2006;31(19, Suppl):S179–S184

10. Yagi M, King AB, Boachie-Adjei O. Incidence, risk factors, and natural course of proximal junctional kyphosis: surgical outcomes review of adult idiopathic scoliosis. Minimum 5 years of follow-up. Spine 2012; 37:1479–1489

11. Bao H, Liu Z, Zhu F, et al. Is the sacro-femoral-pubic angle predictive for pelvic tilt in adolescent idiopathic scoliosis patients? J Spinal Disord Tech 2014; 27:E176–E180

12. Mac-Thiong JM, Transfeldt EE, Mehbod AA, et al. Can c7 plumbline and gravity line predict health related quality of life in adult scoliosis? Spine 2009;34: E519–E527

13. Pfirrmann CW, Metzdorf A, Zanetti M, Hodler J, Boos N. Magnetic resonance classification of lumbar intervertebral disc degeneration. Spine 2001;26:1873–1878

14. Daubs MD, Lenke LG, Bridwell KH, et al. Does correction of preoperative coronal imbalance make a difference in outcomes of adult patients with deformity? Spine 2013;38:476–483

15. Glassman SD, Berven S, Bridwell K, Horton W, Dimar JR. Correlation of radiographic parameters and clinical symptoms in adult scoliosis. Spine 2005;30:682–688

16. Ploumis A, Liu H, Mehbod AA, Transfeldt EE, Winter RB. A correlation of radiographic and functional measurements in adult degenerative scoliosis. Spine 2009;34:1581–1584

17. Cho W, Mason JR, Smith JS, et al. Failure of lumbopelvic fixation after long construct fusions in patients with adult spinal deformity: clinical and radiographic risk factors: clinical article. J Neurosurg Spine 2013;19:445–453

18. Ploumis A, Simpson AK, Cha TD, Herzog JP, Wood KB. Coronal spinal balance in adult spine deformity patients with long spinal fusions: a minimum 2–5 year follow-up study. J Spinal Disord Tech 2013_Sep 27. [Epub ahead of print]

19. Lowe T, Berven SH, Schwab FJ, Bridwell KH. The SRS classification for adult spinal deformity: building on the King/Moe and Lenke classification systems. Spine 2006;31(19, Suppl):S119–S125

20. Bridwell KH. Decision making regarding Smith-Petersen vs. pedicle subtraction osteotomy vs. vertebral column resection for spinal deformity. Spine 2006;31(19, Suppl):S171–S178

21. Toyone T, Shiboi R, Ozawa T, et al. Asymmetrical pedicle subtraction osteotomy for rigid degenerative lumbar kyphoscoliosis. Spine 2012;37:1847–1852

22. Scheer JK, Tang JA, Deviren V, et al. Biomechanical analysis of revision strategies for rod fracture in pedicle subtraction osteotomy. Neurosurgery 2011;69: 164–172, discussion 172

8

Measuring Outcome and Value in Adult Deformity Surgery

Robert Waldrop and Sigurd Berven

Introduction

The definition of a health-related outcome varies in the literature and may encompass a spectrum of measures. Clinical outcome is the end result of health care delivered to patients or populations, and entails such considerations as quality, patient-based assessment, and value of care. Measuring outcomes is complex, and there is no single measure that summarizes the patient's experience, the hospital perspective, the payer perspective, and the treating physician's perspective. Therefore, outcomes must be considered broadly and encompass a spectrum of perspectives and measures. This chapter discusses measures of health-related quality of life (HRQOL), and the application of these measurements in assessing outcomes of spinal deformity surgery.

Outcome measurement is an important aspect of surgeon accountability and is vital in determining the quality and value of health care. Quality may be evaluated based on process measures, objective health outcomes, patient-reported outcome measurements, and cost of care. Value is a broader measure that incorporates an analysis of both quality and cost. This chapter provides an overview of various outcome measures used for spinal deformity, and findings from the literature on outcomes in adult spinal deformity surgery.

Process Measures

Process measures are a reflection of how care is delivered. Examples include compliance with antibiotic or thromboembolic prophylaxis guidelines, the use of surgical "time-outs" before surgery, preoperative risk assessments of patients, and implementing postoperative care protocols for the prevention of common postoperative complications. The utility of process measures depends on how reliably they are linked to clinical outcomes. For example, measuring compliance with preoperative antibiotic guidelines is useful in that it may predict a reduction in the incidence of surgical site infections. Although they are an indirect measure of quality, the implementation and measurement of such guidelines are important in standardizing care and improving quality.

Physiological Outcome Measures

Physiological outcomes represent clinical health metrics that may be measured objectively. In adult spinal deformity, these may include radiographic outcomes, implant survival, and fusion rates. Cobb angle, sagittal vertical axis (SVA), and spinopelvic parameters including pelvic incidence (PI), pelvic tilt (PT), sacral slope (SS), and lumbar lordosis (LL) are all important radiographic measurements in spinal deformity. Although these outcomes are easy to measure and interpret, it is important to evaluate clinical measurements in relation to their correlation with quality measurements (e.g., do radiographic outcomes predict reoperation rates?).

■ Quality Measures

Traditional measurements of quality include outcomes such as operative time and length of hospital stay, as well as rates of complications, reoperations, and readmissions. Such measures provide important information that may be used to compare the performance of individual providers and hospitals and to establish metrics for performance and goals for quality improvement. However, overall quality of care encompasses much more than these traditionally reported quality metrics.

Quality metrics are valuable in identifying outliers, and in improving care processes and pathways. However, overall quality measures are distinct from patient-centered clinical outcome measures. One important concern regarding reliance on quality measures is the possibility that measuring quality alone may lead to a focus on outcomes that are not patient-centered. If the target for outcome were only length of stay or avoidance of readmission, then that goal may incentivize significant undertreatment of complex spinal disorders. **Fig. 8.1** provides an example of a case in which a patient underwent a limited decompression and posterior-based tethering procedure for a complex spinal deformity. Measured by only length of stay or complications of care, the limited decompression surgery would be rated as a high-quality outcome. However, the patient had no improvement in her health status or in her deformity measures. The patient underwent a revision surgery 3 years after the index procedure and was treated with a three-column osteotomy for multiplanar realignment of the spine. The revision surgery resulted in a longer

stay, higher cost, and more risk and potential for complication than the index surgery. However, the patient reported a dramatic improvement in health status that is not captured by the quality metrics alone. It is important to avoid myopic focus on quality metrics without giving priority to patient-centered measures of clinical outcomes in spinal deformity.

■ Patient-Reported Outcomes

Although process measures, physiological outcomes, and traditional quality metrics are important tools for assessing health care quality, they do not reflect the patient's health care experience or the impact of care on HRQOL. There has been an increasing emphasis on patient-based health assessments in recent years. Patient-reported outcome measures (PROMs) may include a spectrum of domains to assess HRQOL. Frequently used domains include disability/functional status, pain and other symptoms, emotional/psychological well-being, general health status, and satisfaction with health care experience. The Visual Analogue Scale (VAS) for pain assessment is another commonly used outcome measure.

Measurement tools for patient-reported outcomes include both disease-specific and general health status measures. Disease-specific measures focus on domains associated with a particular condition or patient population, and have the advantage of increased responsiveness to change (there is a more reliable change in outcome score as the underlying condition changes) compared with general health status measures. Examples of specific outcome tools include the Scoliosis Research Society (SRS-22) questionnaire, the Oswestry Disability Index (ODI), and the Neck Disability Index (NDI).

General health status outcomes tools are advantageous in that they may be used in any patient population and allow for broad comparisons across a spectrum of medical and surgical conditions. However, they are often less responsive to changes in particular conditions or disease states. Examples of generic profiles

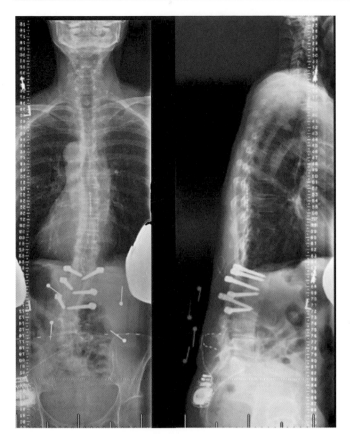

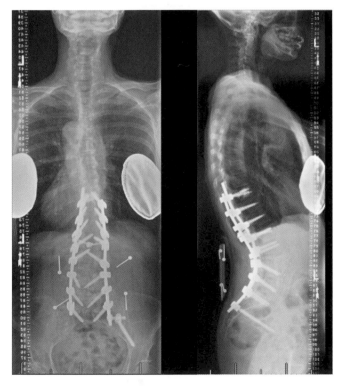

Fig. 8.1a,b **(a)** A 73-year-old woman presented with sagittal and coronal plane deformity, back pain, and neurogenic claudication. She was unable to live independently. The patient was treated with a limited decompression and a posterior-based tethering device. Although the length of stay was 3 days, and there was no complication or readmission within 90 days, there was also no improvement in radiographic or patient-centered clinical outcomes, and the patient remained disabled. **(b)** Postoperative X-rays 2 years after a revision surgery in which the patient was treated with a three-column osteotomy for realignment of the spine. The patient stayed in the hospital for 6 days and her perioperative course was complicated by a supraventricular tachycardia that required cardioversion. At 2-year follow-up, she was living independently and walking without limits.

include the Short Form 36 (SF-36), Short Form 6 Domains (SF-6D), the EuroQOL five dimensions questionnaire (EQ-5D), and the Health Utilities Index (HUI).

Both general health status measures and certain disease-specific outcome tools may be used as indirect measures to calculate utility scores. A utility score reflects societal preferences for a health state. Different health states are rated on a continuous scale from 0 to 1, with the value reflecting a measure of well years of life. Utility scores derived from patient-reported outcome questionnaires using validated instruments provide information on a patient's health status and the value that society places on that health state. Consideration of a utility score over time yields a quality-adjusted life year (QALY), calculated as the utility score multiplied by the number of years that health state is maintained. Thus, the durability of an outcome results in increased QALYs over time. A QALY is an outcome measure that represents a standardized unit for comparison across fields and can be assigned value by society.

◼ Commonly Used Outcome Measurements

The following instruments are commonly used patient-reported outcome measurements in adult spinal deformity that have validated conversions to utility scores/QALYs.

Short Form 36 (SF-36) and Short Form 6 Domains (SF-6D)

The SF-36 is a widely used generic health survey consisting of 36 questions with four physical health scales (physical functioning, physical role limitation, bodily pain, and general health) and four mental health scales (vitality, social functioning, emotional role limitation, and mental health). The SF-6D is an abbreviated version of the SF-36 that has been established as a preference-based health state classification that may be converted to a utility score.[1]

EuroQOL Five Dimensions Questionnaire (EQ-5D)

The EQ-5D is another validated and widely used general health questionnaire that is used to establish a utility score. It includes five health dimensions: mobility, self-care, usual activities, pain/discomfort, and anxiety/depression.

Scoliosis Research Society Questionnaire

The Scoliosis Research Society (SRS) questionnaire measures how spinal deformity affects a patient's HRQOL based on five domains: pain, function, self-image, mental health, and satisfaction. The 22-item questionnaire (SRS-22) is the most widely used and validated version, although several other versions exist (SRS-24, SRS-29, SRS-30). SRS-22 has been validated as a reliable instrument with high internal consistency, responsiveness, reproducibility, and discriminatory capacity for patients with adult deformity.[2,3] A model has been established for translating SRS-22 scores to SF-6D scores to determine utility scores.[4,5]

Oswestry Disability Index (ODI)

The ODI measures HRQOL in patients with low back pain. It rates a patient's disability score based on 10 measures: pain, personal care, sitting, standing, walking, lifting, sleeping, sex life, social life, and traveling. Higher scores correspond to a greater degree of disability. The ODI is a validated and widely used measure that can be reliably translated to a utility score.[6]

◼ Cost and Value

In our current health care economy, cost has become an increasingly important consideration in the assessment of health care interventions. Economic analyses of health care interventions include cost-minimization studies, cost-effectiveness analyses, and cost-utility analyses. An assessment of costs may include direct costs, charges, and reimbursements. Indirect costs such as loss of productivity due to time off from work, transportation to health care facilities, and the cost of caregivers may also be included in cost analyses and incorporate a wider view of total costs from a societal perspective.

Although cost in itself is an important consideration, the value of care provides the most meaningful assessment of a health care intervention. Value of care encompasses both outcome and cost and is defined as the net benefit of care relative to the net cost of care, or what we get for what we spend. The measurement of benefits and costs in spine surgery is not uniform and may vary depending on the perspective of the stakeholder in the health care economy. Hospitals and other health care facilities may emphasize outcomes and costs that affect a single admission such as length of hospital stay, implant utilization, and complications. Third-party payers often focus on outcomes and costs in a medium-term timeframe including readmissions within 90 days or the cost of outpatient care. The value of a health care intervention to the physician and patient is established over a longer timeframe than a single admission; its impact is measured based on HRQOL over a lifetime.

Cost-utility studies provide the most useful information about the value of a health care intervention because a utility score is able to capture a patient's preference for different health states over time. An outcome measure that directly reflects HRQOL and is translatable across disease states, such as QALYs, is an important prerequisite for estimating the value of orthopedic care. The length of follow-up is also an important consideration when measuring value, as the cost of a single episode of care will be significantly discounted by the duration of the benefit.

■ Outcomes of Adult Spinal Deformity Surgery

Several studies have reported various outcomes for the operative and nonoperative management of adult spinal deformity. Estimates of the prevalence of adult spinal deformity in the United States range from 2.5 to 25%[7] However, many of these patients do not seek medical care for their condition, and of those who do, many may have successful management of their symptoms without surgery. Nonoperative care may include physical therapy, core strengthening, weight loss/aerobic activity, pain medications, steroid injections, and alternative modalities such as acupuncture and chiropractic care. For most patients, a trial of nonoperative care should be initiated before surgery is considered. Exceptions include patients with neurologic deficits or significant instability. Surgery may also be indicated in patients with progressive curves, substantial deformity-related pain, and those who have failed appropriate nonoperative treatment. Studies of operative and nonoperative management of adult spinal deformity have demonstrated improved patient-reported outcomes with surgical management.[8–12]

In a review article on adult spinal deformity, Youssef et al[13] summarize the findings of 49 studies reporting outcomes for various surgical strategies including decompression alone versus decompression with fusion; anterior, posterior, or combined surgical approaches; the use of vertebral osteotomies; and levels of instrumented vertebrae. A variety of outcome measurements are reported for each technique.

Radiographic Outcomes

A systematic review of adult scoliosis outcomes by Yadla et al[14] found a range in Cobb angle correction from 9.1 to 53.9 degrees (mean 26.6 degrees, representing an average 40.7% curve correction) in a series of 49 articles published between 1950 and 2009 with minimum 2-year follow-up.

Radiographic outcomes have also been compared between different surgical approaches. Crandall and Revella[15] found no significant difference in coronal curve correction between patients undergoing posterior instrumented fusion in addition to either anterior lumbar interbody fusions (ALIF), with an average correction 69.5%, or transforaminal lumbar interbody fusion (TLIF), with an average correction 68.7%. A literature review by Mundis et al[16] reported improved coronal and sagittal correction with a lateral transpsoas approach compared with open anterior procedures. A retrospective report by Pateder et al[17] comparing patients who underwent posterior only surgery (*n* = 45) versus combined anterior-posterior surgery (*n* = 35) found no significant difference in coronal or sagittal curve correction between the two groups.

Youssef et al[13] also reviewed radiographic outcomes for different types of posterior osteotomies including Smith-Petersen osteotomy (SPO), pedicle subtraction osteotomy (PSO), and vertebral column resection (VCR). These techniques are used to achieve varying degrees of lordosis correction and restoration of sagittal balance. SPO provides the smallest degree of curve correction, achieving up to 10 degrees of lordosis per vertebral level; however, multilevel osteotomies may achieve a large overall correction. Reports of PSO have demonstrated an average 30 degrees of lordotic correction per level. In a comparison of SPO and PSO, Cho et al[18] found an average total correction of 33 degrees for patients undergoing three or more SPOs and 31.7 degrees for patients undergoing PSO, but a significantly lower improvement in sagittal balance for the SPO group than for the PSO group. VCR achieves the highest degree of curve correction. Suk et al[19] reported a mean deformity correction of 59% (109.0 degrees to 45.6 degrees) in 16 patients who underwent posterior VCR. Papadopoulos et al[20] reported that of 45 patients who underwent posterior VCR, the average correction of kyphosis was from 108 degrees to 60 degrees with one patient sustaining a complete spinal cord injury.

Complications

The incidence of complications is an important quality measure in adult spinal deformity. Reported complication rates for spinal deformity surgery are high, but a standardized definition or classification for reporting complications in the literature has not been established. Complication rates have been classified in various

ways, including major versus minor complications, early versus late complications, and surgical versus medical complications. Reported complications in deformity surgery include pseudarthrosis, adjacent segment disease, dural tears, superficial or deep wound infections, implant complications, neurologic deficits, epidural hematoma, wound hematoma, pulmonary embolism, deep vein thrombosis, systemic complications, and death. The incidence of complications may be influenced by patient factors (e.g., age, comorbidities, severity of deformity) or surgical factors (e.g., approach type, need for osteotomy, number of levels fused).

The 49 articles reviewed by Yadla et al[14] report complication rates ranging from 0 to 53%, with a combined total of 897 complications among 2,175 patients (41.2%). Charosky et al[31] reported an overall 39% complication rate among 306 patients over age 50 undergoing adult deformity surgery with either an anterior only, posterior only, or combined approach. Sansur et al[22] reviewed a total of 4,980 cases of adult scoliosis from the SRS morbidity and mortality database and found an overall complication rate of 13.4% and a mortality rate of 0.3%. Significantly higher complication rates resulted from revision surgeries, osteotomies, and combined anterior-posterior surgery.

Youssef et al[13] summarized several studies reporting complication rates of various procedures. Transfeldt et al[23] report a 10% complication rate among adult deformity patients who underwent decompression alone compared with 56% in patients who underwent decompression and fusion. Burneikiene et al[24] reported a 31% incidence of systemic complications and 49% hardware or surgical technique complications in 29 patients undergoing TLIF. Complications of ALIF may include vascular injuries, ilioinguinal and iliohypogastric nerve injuries, damage to the bladder or ureters, pseudarthrosis and subsidence, ileus, lymphocele, and retrograde ejaculation.[13,25] Most of these complications are uncommon, although rates of major and minor complications vary in the literature. In a study of 447 patients, McDonnell et al[26] found a complication rate of 11% for major complications and 24% for minor complications. Complications of the lateral transpsoas approach are often related to manipulation of the lumber plexus. In a prospective multicenter evaluation of 107 adult degenerative scoliosis patients undergoing extreme lateral interbody fusion, Isaacs et al[27] reported a 12.1% major complication rate.

Reoperations

Scheer et al[28] analyzed data from a prospective, multicenter adult spinal deformity database, and examined the rates, indications, timing, and risk factors for reoperation as well as the effect of reoperation on HRQOL measures. In a cohort of 352 patients (268 with at least 1-year follow-up), they found a total reoperation rate of 17%, the majority of which occurred within 1 year of the index operation. The most common indications for reoperation included instrumentation complications and radiographic failure.

There was a 19% reoperation rate for patients undergoing a three-column osteotomy and a 16% reoperation rate for patients not requiring three-column osteotomy; however, three-column osteotomy was not significantly predictive of reoperation at 1 year. The uppermost instrumented vertebra was also not predictive of reoperation. There were no significant differences in the American Society of Anesthesiologists (ASA) grade, Charlson comorbidity index rating, preoperative body mass index (BMI), or smoking history between patients who did not undergo reoperation and those who did. Patients who needed reoperation within 1 year had worse ODI and SRS-22 scores at 1-year follow-up than did patients not needing reoperation. However, there was no significant difference in HRQOL scores at 2 years between patients who required reoperation at 1 year and those who did not.

Other studies have demonstrated similar reoperation rates, ranging from 10 to 21%.[21,29–31] Reasons for revision surgery in adult spinal deformity include pseudarthrosis, curve progression, infection, painful/prominent implants, adjacent segment disease implant failure, and neurologic deficits.[29,30]

HRQOL Outcomes in Adult Spinal Deformity

Despite high complication and reoperation rates in adult spinal deformity surgery, patient satisfaction with these procedures is high. Both condition-specific and general HRQOL outcomes that can be converted to utility scores and compared across the literature are important prerequisites for determining the value of spinal deformity surgery.

Several prospective multicenter studies have demonstrated the benefits of operative treatment of adult spinal deformity compared with nonoperative care in regard to patient-reported health measures including ODI, SRS-22, EQ-5D, and numeric rating scale scores for leg and back pain.[8–12]

Yadla et al[14] reported that in the 49 studies included in their systematic review, ODI and SRS were the most commonly used patient-based outcome instruments, with 11 studies reporting pre- and postoperative ODI scores and 10 studies reporting pre- and postoperative SRS scores. There was an average decrease of 15.7 points (range 3.1–32.3) in ODI score among 911 patients. This improvement in disability outcome correlates with previous reports of significant clinical improvement of ODI scores ranging from 4 to 15 points.[32] Of the 999 patients with pre- and postoperative SRS scores in Yadla et al's review, there was a mean increase in SRS scores of 23.1 points, well above the minimal important difference for SRS scores of 13 points reported by Bagó et al.[33]

Youssef et al[13] summarized the results of studies reporting HRQOL outcomes for patients undergoing various surgical approaches. Crandall and Revella[15] found nonsignificant differences in VAS and ODI outcomes between patients undergoing posterior fusion with either ALIF or TLIF. Mundis et al[16] found significantly improved VAS and ODI scores in a literature review of the lateral approach for adult spinal deformity. Various studies have reported improved patient-reported outcomes following PLIF, including improved ODI, SF-36, and VAS scores.[34–36] Good et al[37] reported similar SRS and ODI scores for both posterior only and combined fusions, with both having improvements at 2-year follow-up.

Cost and Value in Adult Spinal Deformity

Several recent articles have reported on the costs of adult spinal deformity surgery. McCarthy et al[38] studied the total costs of 484 patients undergoing operative treatment of adult spinal deformity with an average follow-up of 4.8 years, and found an average total hospital cost of $120,394. Total cost for primary surgery averaged $103,143, which increased to $111,807 at 1-year follow-up and $126,323 at 4-year follow-up. Hospital readmissions were required in 130 patients (27%), with an average readmission cost of $67,262. Another cost analysis by McCarthy et al[39] found higher direct costs with increasing age, length of hospital stay, length of fusion, and fusions to the pelvis.

Cost-utility studies of adult spinal deformity are lacking in the literature. Although several recently published systematic reviews report on cost-utility analyses in spine care,[40,41] none of the reviewed articles include value assessments in adult deformity. One study by Glassman et al[42] examined the costs and benefits of nonoperative care for adult scoliosis, and questioned the value of nonoperative treatment given their findings of a $10,815 mean treatment cost over a 2-year period with no significant change in HRQOL.

■ Improving Outcomes in Deformity Surgery

Measurement of clinical outcomes and value is an important goal in spine surgery and is critical in establishing accountability for the end result of care. Ernest A. Codman was a surgeon in the early 20th century and a pioneer in advocating outcome measurement and reporting. He proposed an "end results system" in which patients' symptoms, diagnosis, treatment, and outcomes would be tracked over time in an effort to reduce complications and improve qual-

ity of care. At the time, Codman's ideas were seen as radical and met with strong resistance, leading to his dismissal from his faculty position at Massachusetts General Hospital. Although great strides have been made since Codman's time in recognizing the importance of outcome measurement, there is still much room for improvement in the effort to establish regular and reliable systems for outcome measurement and reporting.

There is a high variability in spine surgery with regard to surgical rates, surgical strategies, and costs.[43–45] High variability indicates a lack of consensus on the optimal treatment strategy and a need for further comparative effectiveness research. Reducing variability in spine surgery requires an evidence-based approach to care. The establishment of large multicenter procedural and diagnosis-based registries for spine surgery has been an important step to improving outcome measurement and reporting. These registries provide a reliable system for the reporting of complications, clinical outcomes, and HRQOL outcomes, and facilitate the evaluation of alternative interventions in comparative effectiveness research. With the accurate measurement of complications, quality may be improved through the establishment of clinical protocols based on standards of care in an effort to reduce complications. The widespread use of patient-reported outcome tools that may be translated to a utility score is necessary to address the lack of cost-utility analyses and value-based assessments in adult spinal deformity. An increased emphasis on measuring and improving value in spine care will result in improved outcomes and reduced costs over time. Although we support an effort to reduce variability in spine surgery through an evidence-based approach to care, we also recognize that care is not monolithic, and patient and physician preference must be considered to obtain optimal outcomes.

■ Chapter Summary

Surgical treatment of adult spinal deformity is a high-cost intervention that consistently draws the attention of the lay press and the medical profession due to a perceived lack of effect. In the evolving health care economy, demonstration of value, through cost data coupled with patient-reported outcomes, will be critical in maintaining patient access to care. To best protect our patients' ability to receive care that can effect change in their health status, it is imperative for spinal surgeons to understand and collect patient reported outcomes. Surgical treatment of adult spinal deformity has been shown to have a significant effect on patient-reported outcomes. Although the initial cost of spinal deformity surgery is high, the cost per QALY decreases with increasing durability of the intervention. Thus, it is imperative that we as a profession continue to track and report secondary interventions and complications of care, so that optimal intervention strategies can be created. Determination of appropriate quality metrics and process measures for the delivery of spine care can help achieve improved patient outcomes and potentially lower cost, thus maximizing societal return on investment for the care of adult spinal deformity.

Pearls

- In a value-based health care economy, measures of cost and clinical outcome are important to define cost-effective interventions.
- Patient-centered measures of outcomes provide the most useful assessment of value of interventions in deformity surgery.
- Utility scores are a useful measure of general health status preference that has a definable unit of well-years of life/year.
- Cost per QALY is a measure of value that is sensitive to the magnitude of the health status change and the durability of change.
- Selection of disease-specific, patient-reported outcome should consider validated metrics that can potentially be converted to a utility score.

Pitfalls

- Sole focus on quality metrics and process measures creates a dissociation between interventions and patient-centered outcomes.
- Optimizing quality and process metrics in the absence of patient-centered information may incorrectly guide evidence-based care, and provide incentives for inappropriate care.
- Cost-minimization strategies or focus on cost without regard to effect of treatment on patient reported outcomes will not be a value-optimizing strategy.

References

Five Must-Read References

1. Brazier J, Roberts J, Deverill M. The estimation of a preference-based measure of health from the SF-36. J Health Econ 2002;21:271–292
2. Berven S, Deviren V, Demir-Deviren S, Hu SS, Bradford DS. Studies in the modified Scoliosis Research Society Outcomes Instrument in adults: validation, reliability, and discriminatory capacity. Spine 2003;28:2164–2169, discussion 2169
3. Bridwell KH, Berven S, Glassman S, et al. Is the SRS-22 instrument responsive to change in adult scoliosis patients having primary spinal deformity surgery? Spine 2007;32:2220–2225
4. Bridwell KH, Cats-Baril W, Harrast J, et al. The validity of the SRS-22 instrument in an adult spinal deformity population compared with the Oswestry and SF-12: a study of response distribution, concurrent validity, internal consistency, and reliability. Spine 2005;30:455–461
5. Brazier JE, Roberts J. The estimation of a preference-based measure of health from the SF-12. Med Care 2004;42:851–859

6. Carreon LY, Glassman SD, McDonough CM, Rampersaud R, Berven S, Shainline M. Predicting SF-6D utility scores from the Oswestry disability index and numeric rating scales for back and leg pain. Spine 2009;34:2085–2089
7. United States Bone and Joint Initiative. The Burden of Musculoskeletal Diseases in the United States, 2nd ed. Rosemont, IL: American Academy of Orthopaedic Surgeons; 2011
8. Everett CR, Patel RK. A systematic literature review of nonsurgical treatment in adult scoliosis. Spine 2007;32(19, Suppl):S130–S134
9. Smith JS, Shaffrey CI, Berven S, et al; Spinal Deformity Study Group. Improvement of back pain with operative and nonoperative treatment in adults with scoliosis. Neurosurgery 2009;65:86–93, discussion 93–94
10. Li G, Passias P, Kozanek M, et al. Adult scoliosis in patients over sixty-five years of age: outcomes of operative versus nonoperative treatment at a minimum two-year follow-up. Spine 2009;34:2165–2170

11. Smith JS, Shaffrey CI, Berven S, et al; Spinal Deformity Study Group. Operative versus nonoperative treatment of leg pain in adults with scoliosis: a retrospective review of a prospective multicenter database with two-year follow-up. Spine 2009;34: 1693–1698

12. Bridwell KH, Glassman S, Horton W, et al. Does treatment (nonoperative and operative) improve the two-year quality of life in patients with adult symptomatic lumbar scoliosis: a prospective multicenter evidence-based medicine study. Spine 2009; 34:2171–2178

13. Youssef JA, Orndorff DO, Patty CA, et al. Current status of adult spinal deformity. Global Spine J 2013; 3:51–62

14. Yadla S, Maltenfort MG, Ratliff JK, Harrop JS. Adult scoliosis surgery outcomes: a systematic review. Neurosurg Focus 2010;28:E3

15. Crandall DG, Revella J. Transforaminal lumbar interbody fusion versus anterior lumbar interbody fusion as an adjunct to posterior instrumented correction of degenerative lumbar scoliosis: three year clinical and radiographic outcomes. Spine 2009;34:2126–2133

16. Mundis GM, Akbarnia BA, Phillips FM. Adult deformity correction through minimally invasive lateral approach techniques. Spine 2010;35(26, Suppl): S312–S321

17. Pateder DB, Kebaish KM, Cascio BM, Neubauer P, Matusz DM, Kostuik JP. Posterior only versus combined anterior and posterior approaches to lumbar scoliosis in adults: a radiographic analysis. Spine 2007;32: 1551–1554

18. Cho K-J, Bridwell KH, Lenke LG, Berra A, Baldus C. Comparison of Smith-Petersen versus pedicle subtraction osteotomy for the correction of fixed sagittal imbalance. Spine 2005;30:2030–2037, discussion 2038

19. Suk S-I, Chung E-R, Kim J-H, Kim S-S, Lee J-S, Choi W-K. Posterior vertebral column resection for severe rigid scoliosis. Spine 2005;30:1682–1687

20. Papadopoulos EC, Boachie-Adjei O, Hess WF, et al; Foundation of Orthopedics and Complex Spine, New York, NY. Early outcomes and complications of posterior vertebral column resection. Spine J 2013 Apr 25. [Epub ahead of print]

21. Charosky S, Guigui P, Blamoutier A, Roussouly P, Chopin D; Study Group on Scoliosis. Complications and risk factors of primary adult scoliosis surgery: a multicenter study of 306 patients. Spine 2012;37:693–700

22. Sansur CA, Smith JS, Coe JD, et al. Scoliosis research society morbidity and mortality of adult scoliosis surgery. Spine 2011;36:E593–E597

23. Transfeldt EE, Topp R, Mehbod AA, Winter RB. Surgical outcomes of decompression, decompression with limited fusion, and decompression with full curve fusion for degenerative scoliosis with radiculopathy. Spine 2010;35:1872–1875

24. Burneikiene S, Nelson EL, Mason A, Rajpal S, Serxner B, Villavicencio AT. Complications in patients undergoing combined transforaminal lumbar interbody fusion and posterior instrumentation with deformity correction for degenerative scoliosis and spinal stenosis. Surg Neurol Int 2012;3:25

25. Than KD, Wang AC, Rahman SU, et al. Complication avoidance and management in anterior lumbar interbody fusion. Neurosurg Focus 2011;31:E6

26. McDonnell MF, Glassman SD, Dimar JR II, Puno RM, Johnson JR. Perioperative complications of anterior procedures on the spine. J Bone Joint Surg Am 1996; 78:839–847

27. Isaacs RE, Hyde J, Goodrich JA, Rodgers WB, Phillips FM. A prospective, nonrandomized, multicenter evaluation of extreme lateral interbody fusion for the treatment of adult degenerative scoliosis: perioperative outcomes and complications. Spine 2010;35(26, Suppl):S322–S330

28. Scheer JK, Tang JA, Smith JS, et al; International Spine Study Group. Reoperation rates and impact on outcome in a large, prospective, multicenter, adult spinal deformity database: clinical article. J Neurosurg Spine 2013;19:464–470

29. Pichelmann MA, Lenke LG, Bridwell KH, Good CR, O'Leary PT, Sides BA. Revision rates following primary adult spinal deformity surgery: six hundred forty-three consecutive patients followed-up to twenty-two years postoperative. Spine 2010;35:219–226

30. Kelly MP, Lenke LG, Bridwell KH, Agarwal R, Godzik J, Koester L. Fate of the adult revision spinal deformity patient: a single institution experience. Spine 2013; 38:E1196–E1200

31. Acosta FL Jr, McClendon J Jr, O'Shaughnessy BA, et al. Morbidity and mortality after spinal deformity surgery in patients 75 years and older: complications and predictive factors. J Neurosurg Spine 2011;15: 667–674

32. Fairbank JC, Pynsent PB. The Oswestry Disability Index. Spine 2000;25:2940–2952, discussion 2952

33. Bagó J, Pérez-Grueso FJS, Les E, Hernández P, Pellisé F. Minimal important differences of the SRS-22 Patient Questionnaire following surgical treatment of idiopathic scoliosis. Eur Spine J 2009;18:1898–1904

34. Wu C-H, Wong C-B, Chen L-H, Niu C-C, Tsai T-T, Chen W-J. Instrumented posterior lumbar interbody fusion for patients with degenerative lumbar scoliosis. J Spinal Disord Tech 2008;21:310–315

35. Zimmerman RM, Mohamed AS, Skolasky RL, Robinson MD, Kebaish KM. Functional outcomes and complications after primary spinal surgery for scoliosis in adults aged forty years or older: a prospective study with minimum two-year follow-up. Spine 2010; 35:1861–1866

36. Tsai T-H, Huang T-Y, Lieu A-S, et al. Functional outcome analysis: instrumented posterior lumbar interbody fusion for degenerative lumbar scoliosis. Acta Neurochir (Wien) 2011;153:547–555

37. Good CR, Lenke LG, Bridwell KH, et al. Can posterior-only surgery provide similar radiographic and clinical results as combined anterior (thoracotomy/thoracoabdominal)/posterior approaches for adult scoliosis? Spine 2010;35:210–218

38. McCarthy IM, Hostin RA, Ames CP, et al; International Spine Study Group. Total hospital costs of surgical treatment for adult spinal deformity: an extended follow-up study. Spine J 2014;14:2326–2333

39. McCarthy IM, Hostin RA, O'Brien MF, et al; International Spine Study Group. Analysis of the direct cost of surgery for four diagnostic categories of adult spinal deformity. Spine J 2013;13:1843–1848

40. Indrakanti SS, Weber MH, Takemoto SK, Hu SS, Polly D, Berven SH. Value-based care in the management of spinal disorders: a systematic review of cost-utility analysis. Clin Orthop Relat Res 2012;470:1106–1123

41. Kepler CK, Wilkinson SM, Radcliff KE, et al. Cost-utility analysis in spine care: a systematic review. Spine J 2012;12:676–690

42. Glassman SD, Carreon LY, Shaffrey CI, et al. The costs and benefits of nonoperative management for adult scoliosis. Spine 2010;35:578–582

43. Irwin ZN, Hilibrand A, Gustavel M, et al. Variation in surgical decision making for degenerative spinal disorders. Part I: lumbar spine. Spine 2005;30:2208–2213

44. Sanders JO, Haynes R, Lighter D, et al. Variation in care among spinal deformity surgeons: results of a survey of the Shriners hospitals for children. Spine 2007;32:1444–1449

45. Deyo RA, Mirza SK. Trends and variations in the use of spine surgery. Clin Orthop Relat Res 2006;443:139–146

9

Junctional Issues Following Adult Deformity Surgery

Han Jo Kim, Sravisht Iyer, and Christopher I. Shaffrey, Sr.

■ Introduction

Proximal junctional kyphosis (PJK) was first defined and characterized in the literature by Glattes and colleagues.[1] These authors presented a retrospective series of 81 adult deformity patients and defined abnormal PJK using two criteria: (1) proximal junctional sagittal Cobb angle ≥ 10 degrees (**Fig. 9.1**) and (2) postoperative proximal junctional sagittal Cobb angle at least 10 degrees greater than the preoperative measurement. They reported an incidence of PJK of 26%,[1] and have been supported by subsequent studies reporting rates of PJK ranging from 17 to 61.7%.[2,3] Although PJK is generally asymptomatic, there is a subset of patients (1.4–4%) who present with symptoms requiring further surgery.[4,5]

Risk factors for the development of PJK include advanced age, surgical approach, greater rigidity of construct, greater magnitude of sagittal correction, the presence of preexisting proximal kyphosis, damage to the posterior ligamentous complex, damage to the adjacent facet when instrumenting the upper instrumented vertebra (UIV), fixation to the ilium, type of instrumentation (hooks versus pedicle screws), and the presence of osteoporosis.[1,2,6] Given the large number of identified risk factors, the etiology of PJK is most likely multifactorial in nature. Nonetheless, advanced age is a factor that seems to be uniform across the majority of studies. In addition, the current litera-

ture suggests that PJK may be more prevalent than the rates initially reported 20 years ago.

This chapter synthesizes our current understanding of PJK in adults by reviewing the literature underlying the various etiologies of PJK, discussing the impact of PJK on clinical outcomes, examining the risk factors that lead to revision surgery due to PJK, providing consensus expert opinion on possible methods for minimizing PJK development, and describing indications for surgical treatment.

■ Etiology and Risk Factors for Proximal Junctional Kyphosis

The etiology of PJK is multifactorial and can be divided into surgical, radiographic, and patient-related factors. These are summarized in **Table 9.1.** We will closely examine the literature about these various causes.

Surgical Factors

Disruption of the Posterior Soft Tissues

In their classic paper, Panjabi and White[7] highlighted the role of the posterior spinal ligaments in preventing excessive motion between the vertebrae. Given these ligaments' role as a stabilizer in the spine, the disruption of poste-

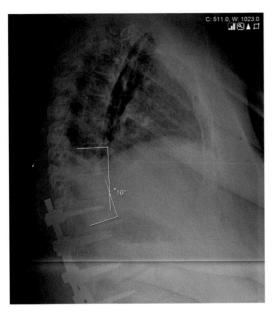
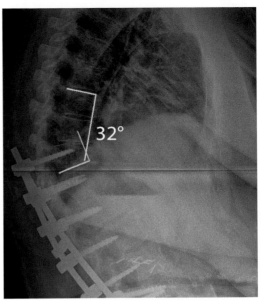

a   b

Fig. 9.1a,b The proximal junctional sagittal Cobb measurement (proximal junctional angle). This is defined as the Cobb angle between the inferior end plate of the upper instrumented vertebra and the superior end plate of the vertebra two levels above.

(a) Postoperative radiograph. **(b)** Radiograph at 6 months that meets both criteria of proximal junctional kyphosis (PJK): proximal junctional angle > 10 degrees and a progression of the proximal junctional angle > 10 degrees.

rior soft tissues has always been viewed as a potential contributor to the development of PJK.

The relative contribution of the posterior soft tissues has been examined in a cadaveric model.[8] The authors of this study performed one of several procedures on motion segments obtained from six human cadavers. These procedures included bilateral transverse hook site preparation, sublaminar hook site preparation, pedicle screw placement, supra- and interspinous ligament transection, and transection of all posterior structures. Following these interventions, the authors measured the torque needed to produce 2.8 degrees of angular displacement, and, based on this measurement, calculated the total flexion stiffness of the motion

Table 9.1 A Summary of Various Risk Factors for PJK Proposed in the Literature

Surgical	Radiographic	Patient-Specific

• Disruption of posterior soft tissues
• Rigidity of instrumentation
• Combined anterior-posterior approach/ fusion
• Upper instrumented vertebrae in the upper thoracic spine
• Fusion to the sacrum
• Degree of correction
  ◦ Increased lumbar lordosis
  ◦ High SVA correction
  ◦ Failure to respect global sagittal alignment
	• Increased preoperative thoracic kyphosis
	• Increased preoperative proximal junctional angle
		• Advanced age
		• High BMI
		• Osteoporosis

Abbreviations: BMI, body mass index; SVA, sagittal vertical axis.

segment. Their data showed that sectioning the supra- and interspinous ligaments led to a significant ($p = 0.02$) loss of flexion stiffness. They found that the posterior ligamentous complex contributed 6.59% to the stiffness of the motion segment and that the stiffness loss could roughly double (12.62%) with the exposure required for placement of instrumentation at the same motion segment.

Similarly, a biomechanical model developed by Cammarata et al[6] showed that complete facetectomy and posterior ligament resection both independently increased the proximal junctional kyphotic angle; combining the two procedures resulted in an even greater increase in the kyphotic angle.

Denis et al[9] presented a series of 67 patients with Scheuermann's kyphosis treated with an instrumented fusion. They highlighted the importance of the posterior ligamentous structures in their series. They separated their cohort of patients with PJK into a group where the fusion stopped short of the proximal end vertebra as well as a group where the proximal end vertebra was included in the fusion. The latter group had three patients who developed PJK. All three were noted to have disruption of the junctional ligamentum flavum with sublaminar hooks or sublaminar wires. In all, the authors noted that disruption of the posterior ligaments was implicated in 25% (5/20) cases of PJK observed in their series.

Although the above findings all hint at the importance of the posterior structures, the true impact of posterior dissection has been difficult to isolate in clinical studies. Although all surgeons would agree that disruption of the muscular, ligamentous, and bony tissue likely occurs cephalad to the UIV, the degree of disruption is difficult to quantify, let alone standardize.[2] Despite this limitation, the spinal reconstructive community generally agrees that damage to the posterior soft tissues likely contributes to the development of PJK.[2]

Rigidity of Instrumentation

In addition to the posterior soft tissues, numerous investigators have commented on the rigidity of instrumentation as a risk factor for development of PJK. This has been a focus in the field, particularly in light of the more rigid, all-pedicle screw constructs that have gained in popularity over the past two decades.

The biomechanical study by Cammarata et al[6] described in the prior section nicely highlights the impact of increasing construct rigidity on the proximal junctional angle. Similarly, Thawrani et al[10] used a porcine cadaver model to show that transverse process hooks provided decreased stiffness compared with an all pedicle screw construct. In the all pedicle screw group, the majority of the motion occurred at the motion segment immediately proximal to the UIV, whereas this transition was more gradual in the transverse process group.

However, clinical studies have not clearly affirmed the findings of the above biomechanical studies.[5,11,12] Y.J. Kim et al[12] found that the use of all pedicle screw constructs was associated with an increased rate of PJK compared with hybrid or hook constructs ($p = 0.04$), but this difference did not remain significant when adjusting for age ($p = 0.33$). Similarly, other published series of adult scoliosis patients have not demonstrated that all pedicle screw constructs were more likely to be associated with PJK than were hybrid screw–hook constructs.[5] Hassanzadeh and colleagues[11] published a series of 47 consecutive adult patients with 2-year follow-up who underwent long spinal fusion with hooks or screws at the UIV. They found no instances of PJK in the 20 patients treated with a hook at the UIV compared with a 29.6% (8/27 patients) rate of PJK in the screws group ($p = 0.01$).

Surgical Approach

Some types of surgical approach have also been associated with PJK. Y.J. Kim and colleagues[12] found that a combined anterior and posterior approach was a risk factor for development of PJK, even when adjusted for age ($p = 0.04$). This finding has been consistently shown to be the case in other series as well.[13,14] In a retrospective series of 249 patients (adults and adolescents) who underwent surgery for idiopathic scoliosis, H.J. Kim et al[14] performed a multivariate analysis to identify risk factors for the development of PJK. They found that patients who underwent an anterior-posterior approach were three times as likely (odds ratio [OR], 3.04; 95% confidence interval [CI], 1.56–5.93) to develop PJK compared with individuals who underwent posterior-only fusion. Additionally, a combined anterior and posterior approach was one of the few factors that could be consistently identified as a risk in a systematic review of the field.[2]

Upper Instrumented Vertebrae

The contribution of the UIV to the development of PJK was suggested in the initial description of the phenomenon. Glattes and colleagues[1] found a significantly higher level of PJK when the instrumentation stopped at T3 (53%) when compared with T4 (12.5%) ($p = 0.02$). A subsequent larger series from the same institution did show that an upper thoracic UIV (T2–6) demonstrated a higher prevalence of PJK (33.67%, 33/98) compared with lower thoracic and upper lumbar UIV ($p = 0.036$).[12] However, this difference did not remain significant when adjusting for age ($p = 0.65$).[12] The UIV, along with a combined anterior-posterior approach, was only one of two independent risk factors associated with the development of PJK in a series of 249 patients.[14]

Bridwell et al[15] found that patients with more advanced PJK (PJK ≥ 20 degrees) were more likely to have a lower number of levels fused (8 versus 11) and were more likely to have a UIV in the lower thoracic spine ($p < 0.001$). Ha et al[16] examined the difference between a UIV in the lower and upper thoracic spine and found that the mechanism of failure was different between the two scenarios. Failure occurred sooner ($p < 0.01$) and was more likely to occur due to fracture in the lower thoracic spine, whereas subluxation was more prevalent in the upper thoracic spine.

Other series, however, failed to identify the UIV as a risk factor for development of PJK.[5,17] A systematic review found low-level evidence that the UIV was among the risk factors associated with the development of PJK.[2]

The mechanism of how the UIV might contribute to the development of PJK is incompletely understood. Proposed theories include both damage to the adjacent facet joint that can occur more easily in the upper thoracic spine[18] as well as the interface between the mobile cervical and relatively static thoracic spine.[1]

Instrumentation to the Sacrum/Ilium

In cases of adult scoliosis, extension of the fusion to the sacropelvis and the subsequent increase in stiffness of the construct has been thought to contribute to the development of PJK. In their series of adult patients, Y.J. Kim and colleagues[12] found a higher rate of PJK in patients whose lower instrumented vertebra (LIV) was S1 compared with patients with an LIV of L5 or above (51% vs 30%, $p = 0.009$). This remained a strong trend ($p = 0.059$) even after adjusting for age. Yagi et al[5] observed a similar trend; in their series, fusion to the sacrum was associated with a significantly higher incidence of PJK (an increase of 27.6%, $p = 0.02$). A more recent clinical series also found that patients with PJK requiring revision were more likely to have fusions extending to the pelvis (74% vs 91%, $p = 0.02$).[19] Fusion to the sacrum was also associated with an increased risk of progression of PJK to greater than 20 degrees.[15]

Magnitude of Correction

More recently, as we have begun to understand the importance of global sagittal alignment, investigators have sought to determine if parameters of sagittal alignment correlate with the incidence of PJK. In general, studies have found that an increase in sagittal balance correction and an increase in lumbar lordosis correlate with the development of PJK.[5,17,19,20] The mechanism underlying this increased rate of PJK is unknown. In their retrospective series, H.J. Kim et al[19] found that patients requiring revision surgery for PJK had a lumbar lordosis (LL) that was closer to the pelvic incidence (PI), whereas those without PJK had a LL much lower than PI. Their findings are similar to those of Maruo and colleagues,[17] who showed that increasing LL more than 30 degrees was associated with a significantly higher incidence of PJK (58% vs 28%, $p = 0.003$).

Similarly, patients requiring revision surgery with PJK had a lower postoperative sagittal vertical axis (SVA) (0.8 vs 4.1 cm) and a higher magnitude of SVA correction (9 vs 4 cm) compared with those without PJK.[19] These findings are generally in keeping with those of Yagi and colleagues,[5] who saw that a SVA correction greater than 5 cm led to a 50% incidence of PJK ($p = 0.01$). Another series of 54 patients demonstrated that the risk of PJK decreases by 30% for every centimeter increase in the C7-plumbline.[20] In the same series, the C7-plumbline had returned closer to its preoperative position in all patients by final follow-up (average 2.23 years).

The interplay between thoracic kyphosis and lumbar lordosis, that is, the global sagittal alignment (GSA), is also becoming an increasingly important concept in understanding PJK. In the same study where they looked at sagittal correction, Yagi and colleagues[5] showed that a nonideal postoperative GSA (thoracic kyphosis [TK] + LL + PI > 45°) led to a 70% rate of PJK ($p < 0.001$). Maruo et al[17] also showed that ideal global sagittal alignment protected against the development of PJK. The importance of spinal balance is also highlighted by Mendoza-Lattes and colleagues,[20] who found that the difference between TK and LL was inversely proportional to the risk of developing PJK.

Taken together, these studies add to our growing understanding of global sagittal balance. They suggest that the goal of restoring the SVA to 0 cm may not be optimal for all patients. Indeed, studies of asymptomatic volunteers have consistently shown increased age to be correlated with greater SVA.[21,22] They also highlight the need for further studies to establish the optimal spinopelvic parameters for surgeons to target (i.e., to understand the difference between LL + 9° and LL – 9°).[19]

Radiographic Factors

Preoperative Thoracic Kyphosis

High preoperative TK may predispose to PJK in both adult and pediatric populations. In the adult population, Maruo and colleagues[17] showed that preoperative TK greater than 30 degrees was a risk factor for developing PJK (62% vs 29%, $p = 0.002$). Similarly, Mendoza-Lattes and colleagues[20] found that patients with PJK had a larger difference between TK and LL at baseline ($p = 0.012$). These patients also presented with lower sacral slope and signs of pelvic retroversion.

Proximal Junctional Angle

Lee and colleagues,[23] one of the first groups to describe PJK in patients with idiopathic scoliosis, found that a preoperative PJ angle greater than 5 degrees was a risk factor for development of subsequent junctional kyphosis. This work has been supported by Denis et al's[9] series of Scheuermann patients. The large majority of cases of PJK observed in that series were noted when the proximal extent of the fusion did not include the kyphotic proximal end vertebra. Maruo and colleagues[17] were able to demonstrate that a proximal junctional angle (PJA) greater than 10 degrees ($p = 0.016$), in addition to a PI > 55° ($p = 0.037$), was a risk factor for the development of PJK.[17]

Patient Factors

Patient-specific factors such as advanced age, high body mass index (BMI), the presence of osteoporosis, smoking, and the presence of other comorbidities are always important to consider prior to spine surgery. Not surprisingly, many of these factors have been linked to the development of PJK. In the adult literature, increasing age has been associated with the incidence of PJK and PJK requiring revision in numerous case series.[1,2,15,19,24]

Interestingly, the link between high BMI and the development of PJK is less clear in the literature. Bridwell et al[15] were able to show that higher BMI ($p = 0.015$) and the presence of a comorbidity ($p = 0.001$) were associated with the development of PJ angle > 20 degrees. However, other series from the same institution have failed to show the same link between high BMI and PJK (defined in the traditional manner using 10 degrees as a cutoff).[19,24]

Given that a large proportion of PJK occurs due to fracture at the UIV,[17] it is not surprising that osteoporosis plays a critical role in the development of PJK. In one series, osteoporotic patients over the age of 65 who underwent a minimum five-level fusion were found to have pedicle and compression fractures at a rate of 13%, with PJK occurring in 26% of patients.[25] In a small series of 10 adult patients, Watanabe and colleagues[26] found that osteopenia and preoperative comorbidities were common among patients with proximal vertebral fracture and subluxation. Case series in adult patients have found that osteoporosis is much more prevalent in individuals with PJK than in those without.[24]

Timing of Proximal Junctional Kyphosis

The majority of the cases of PJK are identified within the first year postoperatively.[5,14] The patients who do go on to develop PJK progress to about one half (53%) of their total degree of PJK by 3 months.[5] Similarly, Y.J. Kim and colleagues[12] reported that 59% of progression of the PJA occurs within the first 8 weeks. Maruo et al[17] reported that 62% of cases with PJK were identified within 8 weeks, with fracture being the most common cause.

Clinical Outcomes After Proximal Junctional Kyphosis

Clinical outcomes after PJK are summarized in **Table 9.2**. In general, most studies have shown that most cases of PJK are asymptomatic, and that this condition does not substantially alter clinical outcome. There are, however, two recent series that do show that patients with PJK have increased pain levels compared with those patients without PJK.[19,24] The difference in pain levels between the two groups met the minimal clinically important difference.[24] The incidence of symptomatic pain (i.e., upper back

pain reported by the patient at follow-up) was also markedly higher in the group with PJK (29.4% vs 0.9%, $p < 0.001$). These more recent results highlight the importance of furthering our understanding of PJK; as we shall see in the following sections, the early descriptions of PJK as a radiographic finding that warrants follow-up might be understating the true impact of the condition.

Investigators are now turning a closer eye to the concept of symptomatic PJK to see how these cases might impact clinical outcomes. Yagi and colleagues[5] found that their patients with symptomatic PJK had a significantly higher Oswestry Disability Index (ODI) score compared with patients without PJK.[5] Similarly, H.J. Kim et al[19] found lower ODI and pain scores in patients with PJK and lower pain scores in patients undergoing revision for PJK. Importantly, they found lower outcomes across all domains of the *Scoliosis Research Society* (SRS) questionnaire in patients with PJK, though these outcomes did not reach statistical significance.

Revision Surgery for Proximal Junctional Kyphosis

The majority of cases of PJK are asymptomatic and do not require intervention. Reported rates of revision due to PJK have ranged from 1.4 to 11.2% with pain being the most common reason for revision.[4,19,27,28]

Severe cases of PJK can lead to significant sagittal imbalance and disability. In a small series of 10 patients, Watanabe et al[26] reported vertebral subluxation and severe neurologic deficit in two of their 10 patients as a result of progression of PJK.

Hart et al[28] reported on a case series from the *Invasive Species Specialist Group* (ISSG) database. Their definition of proximal junctional failure (PJF) was "severe PJK," which was further defined as a change of more than 10 degrees of kyphosis between the UIV and the vertebra two levels above the UIV (UIV +2), along with one or more of the following: fracture of the

Table 9.2 Clinical Outcomes for PJK that Have Been Reported in the Literature*

Study	Patient Demographics and Follow-Up	Outcomes Scales and Reported Change		PJK	No PJK	P value
Y.J. Kim et al[12]	N = 161 Age: mean 45.2 years (range, 18.1–73.0) Follow-up: min 5 years, avg 7.8 years PJK rate: 39%	SRS-24	Total	77 ± 18.4	79 ± 19.3	0.47
			Pain	17 ± 5.9	18 ± 6.0	0.70
			Self-image	19 ± 4.0	19 ± 4.3	0.74
			Function	17 ± 5.2	18 ± 4.6	0.70
			Satisfaction	9 ± 1.9	9 ± 1.5	0.84
H.J. Kim et al[24]	N = 364** Age: PJK, 53.3 ± 14.5 years; no PJK, 48.9 ± 15.0 years Follow-up: 3.5 years (range, 2–6) PJK rate: 39.5%	Change in ODI Change in SRS domain Symptomatic pain	Δ ODI	−14.7 ± 16.8	−14.4 ± 16.3	0.862
			Δ Activity	0.4 ± 0.8	0.5 ± 0.7	0.09
			Δ Self-image	1.2 ± 0.9	1.0 ± 0.8	0.12
			Δ Mental	0.2 ± 0.8	0.2 ± 0.8	0.73
			Δ Pain	0.8 ± 1.1	1.2 ± 1.0	0.04
			Sympt. pain	29.4%	0.9%	< 0.001
Yagi et al[5]	N = 76 Age: mean 48.8 years (range, 23–75) Follow-up: 5.3 years (2–16) PJK rate: 26% Symptomatic PJK: 5.26%	ODI SRS-22r	ODI	23.8 ± 18.6	24.3 ± 12.9	0.46
			SRS total	3.67 ± 0.62	3.86 ± 0.75	0.10
			Function	2.98 ± 0.81	3.31 ± 0.75	0.07
			Pain	3.66 ± 0.89	3.86 ± 0.75	0.34
			Self-image	3.88 ± 0.78	4.03 ± 0.73	0.49
			Mental	3.94 ± 0.56	3.87 ± 0.73	0.62
			Satisfaction	4.29 ± 0.69	4.45 ± 0.66	0.72
			ODI	53.0 ± 15.6†	24.3 ± 12.9	< 0.001
			SRS total	3.30 ± 0.69†	3.86 ± 0.75	0.26
			Function	3.00 ± 0.72†	3.31 ± 0.75	0.13
			Pain	3.39 ± 0.91†	3.86 ± 0.75	0.77
			Self-image	3.53 ± 0.31†	4.03 ± 0.73	0.33
			Mental	3.23 ± 0.31†	3.87 ± 0.73	0.94
			Satisfaction	3.23 ± 0.81†	4.45 ± 0.66	0.66

H.J. Kim et al[19]	N = 206 Age: No PJK, mean 49.9 years; PJK, mean 51.3 years Revision PJK, mean 60.1 years Follow-up: 3.5 years (minimum 2 years) PJK rate (revision + no revision): 34% PJK requiring revision: 10.7%	ODI SRS-22r	*ODI* Activity Self-image Mental *Pain* Satisfaction	29.1 ± 18.2¶ 3.4 ± 0.9¶ 3.6 ± 0.8¶ 3.5 ± 0.9¶ 3.7 ± 0.9¶ 4.0 ± 0.9¶	*22.65 ± 17.8* *0.04* 3.61 ± 0.87 0.15 3.79 ± 0.78 0.22 3.74 ± 0.81 0.20 *4.02 ± 0.95* *0.04* 4.08 ± 0.83 0.38
			ODI Activity Self-image Mental *Pain* Satisfaction	30.7 ± 20.6§ 3.5 ± 0.6§ 3.9 ± 0.7§ 4.0 ± 0.8§ 3.5 ± 0.9§ 3.0 ± 0.6§	22.65 ± 17.8 0.73 3.61 ± 0.87 0.29 3.79 ± 0.78 0.66 3.74 ± 0.81 0.13 *4.02 ± 0.95* *0.04* 4.08 ± 0.83 0.06

Abbreviations: ODI, Oswestry Disability Index; SRS, Scoliosis Research Society scale; Δ, change.

Note. More recent studies have suggested that perhaps PJK causes more symptomatic upper back pain and could lead to lower functional outcomes.

*Sigificant findings are italicized.

**The number of patients that had functional outcomes differs from the total number of patients that met the inclusion criteria. For ODI, n = 182/220 non-PJK group, 122/144 PJK group. For SRS, n = 184–189/220 (varies by subscale) for the non-PJK group and 121–125/144 (varies by subscale) for the PJK group.

†Outcomes in patients with symptomatic PJK (n = 4). These outcomes were reported separately from patients with asymptomatic PJK.

¶Outcomes in patients with PJK not requiring revision (n = 48), p values compared with patients with no PJK.

§Outcomes for patients requiring revision (n = 22), p values compared with patients with no PJK.

vertebral body of UIV or UIV +1, posterior osseoligamentous disruption, or pullout of instrumentation at the UIV. In their series, they identified 57 patients from a series of 1,218 consecutive adult patients who met this definition of PJF (4.68%). Of the 57 cases of PJF, 27 (47.4%) underwent revision surgery within 6 months of their index operation. Of the causes of PJF, fracture was the most common (56%), followed by soft tissue failure (35%) and screw pullout (9%). Of the risk factors identified for revision surgery, a combined anterior/posterior approach ($p = 0.001$) and higher PJK angulation ($p = 0.034$) were found to be significant. Of the various modes of failure, only the presence of traumatic mechanism of failure, which occurred in six patients, was deemed to predispose patients to a revision ($p = 0.019$). A higher SVA also trended toward being a significant predictor of revision ($p = 0.090$) along with female sex ($p = 0.066$). The overall rate of revision surgery was 2.21%.

A similar study was conducted by Yagi and colleagues[4] as part of the Complex Spine Study Group. They utilized a consecutive series of 1,668 patients treated for adult spinal deformity and greater than five levels of fusion. Their series had longer follow-up (2 to 12 year, mean 4.3 years), and they also focused on patients older than 50 at the time of surgery. They defined PJF as PJK requiring revision and identified 23 patients (1.4%). The large majority of these 23 patients (17 patients, 74%) had been revision surgery cases at the time of their long segment fusion and all had received posterior pedicle screw constructs. Osteopenia was prevalent (10/23, 43%), but, interestingly, none of these patients had osteoporosis. Sixteen patients were revised for intolerable pain, another six for a neurologic deficit, and one for head ptosis. The authors found that a majority of these failures occurred early, with a mean time to PJF (revision) of 10.5 ± 9.3 months; 87% had been revised within 2 years of surgery. H.J. Kim et al[19] reported that a higher lumber lordosis and an increased SVA correction are risk factors for revision due to PJK. They reported a revision rate of 10.7%.

Moving forward, important work remains to be done regarding our understanding of PJF.

A classification system for PJK and a clear definition of PJF are needed before we progress toward defining the risk factors for PJF. Additionally, the optimal magnitude of correction also remains to be determined.

Preventing Proximal Junctional Kyphosis

To date, no definitive methods have been described to prevent PJK, although several approaches have been suggested. Two studies have reported on technical tricks to reduce the incidence of PJK.[11,29,30] Hassanzadeh et al[11] found no instances of PJK in 20 patients treated with a hook at the UIV compared with a 29.6% (8/27 patients) rate of PJK in patients who were treated with a pedicle screw at the UIV ($p = 0.01$). Additionally, they found that patients with hooks had significantly higher functional scores compared with those with screws ($p < 0.01$). These data have not been replicated to date.

Given that vertebral fractures represent a common etiology for PJK and PJF, investigators have also studied the impact of prophylactic one- and two-level vertebroplasty above long fusions. Results reported include both biomechanical[29] and clinical[30] data. In a biomechanical model using 18 cadaveric spines, Kebaish et al[29] were able to show a significant reduction in vertebral compression fractures when two-level vertebroplasty (UIV and UIV +1) was compared with one-level (UIV only) or no vertebroplasty. A clinical series from the same group followed 38 patients with two-level vertebroplasty (UIV and UIV +1) for 2 years.[30] They reported a lower rate of PJK or PJF (PJK 8%, PJF 5%, combined 13%) than previously published rates. Their study did not include a control cohort (i.e., patients who had not received vertebroplasty), and did not show any significant differences in clinical outcomes between the groups with and without PJK or PJF.

Finally, Yanik et al[31] reported on a series of 60 patients treated for Scheuermann kyphosis. To reduce the stiffness of the proximal construct, they studied the impact of leaving two screw threads out of the posterior cortex when placing pedicle screws at the UIV. They theorized that this would reduce the stiffness at the proximal aspect of the construct. At an average of 2-year follow-up, they found that the screws with threads left out of the cortex had a lower PJ angle (4.44 ± 1.55 degrees vs 8.08 ± 2.96 degrees) when compared with standard pedicle screw insertion (p = 0.001). This group also had no cases of PJK, compared with a 17.2% (5/29, p = 0.02) rate with the standard screw technique. Finally, they were also able to show an improvement in the physical component of the Short Form 36 score in the group treated with the modified screw insertion.

Revision Strategies

The approach to the patient with PJK is similar to the approach to the patient with other sagittal plane deformities. Our indications for a revision operation are as follows:

1. Progressive deformity
2. Pain that has failed nonoperative measures for management
3. Implant prominence with imminent skin breakdown
4. Neurologic deficit or cord compression

The decision about the UIV level selection is based on several factors, but generally speaking, PJK cases with a UIV in the lower thoracic spine should be extended up to the upper thoracic spine, and cases with a UIV in the upper thoracic spine should be extended up to T1–2 or into the cervical spine.

Osteotomies may also be necessary in the treatment of PJK. Osteotomy selection is based on the rigidity of PJK. Flexible PJK (**Fig. 9.2**) can usually be treated without an osteotomy, or with a posterior column only osteotomy (**Fig. 9.2d**), whereas rigid deformities (**Fig. 9.3**) may necessitate a three-column osteotomy (i.e., pedicle subtraction osteotomy or vertebral column resection) (**Fig. 9.3c**). Flexibility can be assessed with hyperextension or supine radiographs as well as the scout images on some computed tomography (CT) scans (as long as a head support was not used during the scan).

For cases where a neurologic deficit or symptomatic cord compression is present, a vertebral column resection may be necessary to decompress the kyphotic area where the cord compression is likely to be present. Anatomic realignment is essential to relieve the cord compression.

The goal for the revision operation should avoid the temptation for overcorrection; instead, the goal should be an SVA close to 4 to 5 cm. Overcorrection can lead to a recurrence of PJK and necessitate additional operations and unnecessary risk for patients.

■ Chapter Summary

Proximal junctional kyphosis is defined using two criteria: (1) proximal junctional sagittal Cobb angle ≥ 10 degrees, and (2) postoperative proximal junctional sagittal Cobb angle at least 10 degrees greater than the preoperative measurement.[1] PJK is generally an early postoperative phenomenon, and most cases typically are recognized in the first year after surgery.[5,14] Rates of PJK reported in the literature range from 17 to 61.7%.[2,3]

Proximal junctional kyphosis is likely multifactorial in origin. Risk factors for the development of PJK can be categorized as surgical, radiographic, and patient-related factors. Advanced age appears to be the most important patient-related risk factor. Surgical risk factors to consider include greater magnitude of sagittal correction, damage to the adjacent facet when instrumenting the UIV, damage to the posterior ligamentous complex, a combined anterior and posterior approach, fixation to the ilium, and certain types of instrumentation. Of the above, the magnitude of correction is particularly important, as an SVA of 0 cm may not be optimal for all patients.[21,22] A higher postoperative LL and an SVA correction of greater than 5 cm have both been associated with the development of PJK.[17,19] To date, no definitive methods have been described to prevent PJK. Some investigators have described technical tricks to reduce the incidence of PJK.[11,31]

Patients with PJK are generally asymptomatic. However, recent studies have shown that these patients may have increased pain levels and worse functional outcome measures.[19,24]

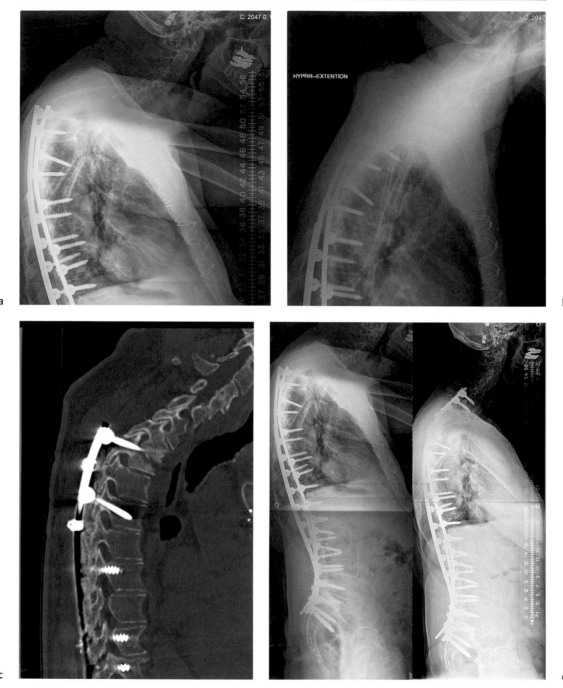

Fig. 9.2a–d A patient presenting with PJK who was treated with extension of the posterior fusion and posterior osteotomies only. **(a)** Lateral radiograph. **(b)** Hyperextension view, clearly showing a flexible deformity. **(c)** Computed tomography (CT) scan. **(d)** Preoperative *(left)* and postoperative *(right)* standing radiographs.

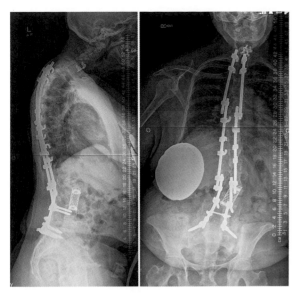

Fig. 9.3a–c A patient with a rigid deformity. **(a)** Preoperative images of the proximal kyphotic deformity. **(b)** CT scan and recumbent film show a solid fusion extending up to the upper instrumented vertebra (UIV) with a rigid deformity. This patient required a three-column osteotomy to correct the PJK. **(c)** Pre- and postrevision radiographs.

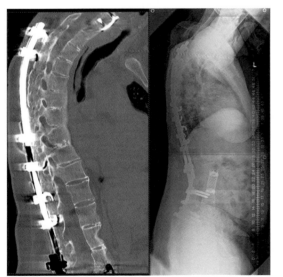

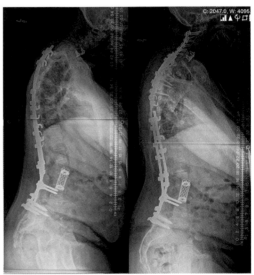

In the subset of patients who are symptomatic, pain is the most common complaint and the most common reason for revision. Reported rates for revision for PJK range from 1.2 to 11.4%.[4,19,27,28] Patients requiring revision for PJK are generally approached similarly to patients with other sagittal plane deformities. Osteotomies may be necessary and are chosen based on the rigidity of the PJK. When revising PJK, the temptation for overcorrection should be avoided.

Pearls

- The appropriate magnitude of correction and global sagittal alignment are critical to achieving successful outcomes and avoiding the development of PJK. An SVA of 4 cm is a reasonable goal, especially for those patients over 60 years of age.
- Proximal junctional kyphosis is an early postoperative phenomenon, and most cases can typically be observed within 2 to 6 months postoperatively. Similarly, cases of junctional failure typically are evident within the first year.
- When revising cases of PJK, it is crucial to consider the rigidity of the deformity, as flexible PJK may be treated with instrumentation and fusion only, without an osteotomy or posterior column osteotomies only.

Pitfalls

- Careful attention must be paid to global sagittal alignment; attempting to aggressively correct all patients to an SVA of 0 cm has been shown to predispose patients to PJK.
- Although no consensus exists on preventing PJK, surgeons must pay close attention to the integrity of the posterior soft tissues and the rigidity of the construct, and must select an appropriate UIV. Failure to consider these factors may lead to the development of PJK.
- Although most cases of PJK are asymptomatic, these patients may have increased pain and worse functional scores. They must be followed regularly to ensure stable kyphosis and acceptable outcomes.

References
Five Must-Read References

1. Glattes RC, Bridwell KH, Lenke LG, Kim YJ, Rinella A, Edwards C II. Proximal junctional kyphosis in adult spinal deformity following long instrumented posterior spinal fusion: incidence, outcomes, and risk factor analysis. Spine 2005;30:1643–1649
2. Kim HJ, Lenke LG, Shaffrey CI, Van Alstyne EM, Skelly AC. Proximal junctional kyphosis as a distinct form of adjacent segment pathology after spinal deformity surgery: a systematic review. Spine 2012;37(22, Suppl):S144–S164
3. Lee JH, Kim JU, Jang JS, Lee SH. Analysis of the incidence and risk factors for the progression of proximal junctional kyphosis following surgical treatment for lumbar degenerative kyphosis: minimum 2-year follow-up. Br J Neurosurg 2014;28:252–258
4. Yagi M, Rahm M, Gaines R, et al; Complex Spine Study Group. Characterization and surgical outcomes of proximal junctional failure in surgically treated patients with adult spinal deformity. Spine 2014;39: E607–E614
5. Yagi M, King AB, Boachie-Adjei O. Incidence, risk factors, and natural course of proximal junctional kyphosis: surgical outcomes review of adult idiopathic scoliosis. Minimum 5 years of follow-up. Spine 2012;37:1479–1489
6. Cammarata M, Aubin CE, Wang X, Mac-Thiong JM. Biomechanical risk factors for proximal junctional kyphosis: a detailed numerical analysis of surgical instrumentation variables. Spine 2014;39:E500– E507
7. Panjabi MM, White AA III. Basic biomechanics of the spine. Neurosurgery 1980;7:76–93
8. Anderson AL, McIff TE, Asher MA, Burton DC, Glattes RC. The effect of posterior thoracic spine anatomical structures on motion segment flexion stiffness. Spine 2009;34:441–446
9. Denis F, Sun EC, Winter RB. Incidence and risk factors for proximal and distal junctional kyphosis following surgical treatment for Scheuermann kyphosis: minimum five-year follow-up. Spine 2009;34:E729– E734
10. Thawrani DP, Glos DL, Coombs MT, Bylski-Austrow DI, Sturm PF. Transverse process hooks at upper instrumented vertebra provide more gradual motion transition than pedicle screws. Spine 2014;39:E826– E832
11. Hassanzadeh H, Gupta S, Jain A, El Dafrawy M, Skolasky RL, Kebaish KM. Type of anchor at the proximal fusion level has a significant effect on the incidence of proximal junctional kyphosis and outcome in adults after long posterior spinal fusion. Spine Deformity 2013;1:299–305
12. Kim YJ, Bridwell KH, Lenke LG, Glattes CR, Rhim S, Cheh G. Proximal junctional kyphosis in adult spinal deformity after segmental posterior spinal instrumentation and fusion: minimum five-year follow-up. Spine 2008;33:2179–2184
13. Wang J, Zhao Y, Shen B, Wang C, Li M. Risk factor analysis of proximal junctional kyphosis after posterior fusion in patients with idiopathic scoliosis. Injury 2010;41:415–420
14. Kim HJ, Yagi M, Nyugen J, Cunningham ME, Boachie-Adjei O. Combined anterior-posterior surgery is the most important risk factor for developing proximal junctional kyphosis in idiopathic scoliosis. Clin Orthop Relat Res 2012;470:1633–1639
15. Bridwell KH, Lenke LG, Cho SK, et al. Proximal junctional kyphosis in primary adult deformity surgery:

evaluation of 20 degrees as a critical angle. Neurosurgery 2013;72:899–906

16. Ha Y, Maruo K, Racine L, et al. Proximal junctional kyphosis and clinical outcomes in adult spinal deformity surgery with fusion from the thoracic spine to the sacrum: a comparison of proximal and distal upper instrumented vertebrae. J Neurosurg Spine 2013;19:360–369

17. Maruo K, Ha Y, Inoue S, et al. Predictive factors for proximal junctional kyphosis in long fusions to the sacrum in adult spinal deformity. Spine 2013;38: E1469–E1476

18. Helgeson MD, Shah SA, Newton PO, et al; Harms Study Group. Evaluation of proximal junctional kyphosis in adolescent idiopathic scoliosis following pedicle screw, hook, or hybrid instrumentation. Spine 2010;35:177–181

19. Kim HJ, Bridwell KH, Lenke LG, et al. Patients with proximal junctional kyphosis requiring revision surgery have higher postoperative lumbar lordosis and larger sagittal balance corrections. Spine 2014;39: E576–E580

20. Mendoza-Lattes S, Ries Z, Gao Y, Weinstein SL. Proximal junctional kyphosis in adult reconstructive spine surgery results from incomplete restoration of the lumbar lordosis relative to the magnitude of the thoracic kyphosis. Iowa Orthop J 2011;31:199–206

21. Vedantam R, Lenke LG, Keeney JA, Bridwell KH. Comparison of standing sagittal spinal alignment in asymptomatic adolescents and adults. Spine 1998;23: 211–215

22. Gelb DE, Lenke LG, Bridwell KH, Blanke K, McEnery KW. An analysis of sagittal spinal alignment in 100 asymptomatic middle and older aged volunteers. Spine 1995;20:1351–1358

23. Lee GA, Betz RR, Clements DH III, Huss GK. Proximal kyphosis after posterior spinal fusion in patients with idiopathic scoliosis. Spine 1999;24:795–799

24. Kim HJ, Bridwell KH, Lenke LG, et al. Proximal junctional kyphosis results in inferior SRS pain subscores in adult deformity patients. Spine 2013;38:896–901

25. DeWald CJ, Stanley T. Instrumentation-related complications of multilevel fusions for adult spinal deformity patients over age 65: surgical considerations and treatment options in patients with poor bone quality. Spine 2006;31(19, Suppl):S144–S151

26. Watanabe K, Lenke LG, Bridwell KH, Kim YJ, Koester L, Hensley M. Proximal junctional vertebral fracture in adults after spinal deformity surgery using pedicle screw constructs: analysis of morphological features. Spine 2010;35:138–145

27. Reames DL, Kasliwal MK, Smith JS, Hamilton DK, Arlet V, Shaffrey CI. Time to development, clinical and radiographic characteristics, and management of proximal junctional kyphosis following adult thoracolumbar instrumented fusion for spinal deformity. J Spinal Disord Tech 2014

28. Hart R, McCarthy I, O'Brien M, et al. Identification of decision criteria for revision surgery among patients with proximal junctional failure after surgical treatment of spinal deformity. Spine 2013;38:E1223–E1227

29. Kebaish KM, Martin CT, O'Brien JR, LaMotta IE, Voros GD, Belkoff SM. Use of vertebroplasty to prevent proximal junctional fractures in adult deformity surgery: a biomechanical cadaveric study. Spine J 2013; 13:1897–1903

30. Martin CT, Skolasky RL, Mohamed AS, Kebaish KM. Preliminary results of the effect of prophylactic vertebroplasty on the incidence of proximal junctional complications after posterior spinal fusion to the low thoracic spine. Spine Deformity 2013;1:132–138

31. Yanik HS, Ketenci IE, Polat A, et al. Prevention of proximal junctional kyphosis after posterior surgery of Scheuermann kyphosis: An operative technique. J Spinal Disord Tech 2014 Jul 29. [Epub ahead of print]

10

Biomechanics and Material Science for Deformity Correction

Manabu Ito, Yuichiro Abe, and Remel Alingalan Salmingo

■ Introduction

The first application of a metallic implant to the human spine was reported by Hadra[1] in 1891. Silver wires were placed in the thoracic spine for treatment of a spinal fracture. The most important historical event in spinal reconstruction surgery was the invention of the Harrington instrumentation in the middle of the 20th century.[2] Paul Harrington developed these spinal implants, consisting of hooks and rods made of stainless steel, for treatment of severe spinal deformity and fracture-dislocations of the spine. Since the introduction of his device, surgeries to correct and stabilize the spine with metallic implants have undergone dramatic development, and surgeries using metallic implants to correct and stabilize the damaged spine became known as spinal instrumentation surgery. The Harrington instrumentation surgery was modified by his successors, who added sublaminar wires, tapes, and pedicle screws.[3] Since 2000, pedicle screws and rods have been widely used for spinal deformity surgery due to their biomechanical superiority. Of the biomaterials used for spinal deformity surgery, titanium alloys are the most popular material at the present time due to their improved biocompatibility and because they entail fewer metal-related artifacts in magnetic resonance imaging (MRI).[4] Historically, stainless steel and cobalt-chromium (Co-Cr) were discovered much earlier than titanium alloys (**Table 10.1**). Spinal implants made of stainless steel or Co-Cr are currently used for patients with rigid spinal curves due to their superior mechanical properties to titanium alloys.

There is no consensus on how to select metallic materials for spinal deformity correction today, and spine surgeons depend on their personal experience through their medical career. This chapter discusses metallic spinal implants and the biomechanics of the deformity correction of the spine. It is imperative that practitioners be familiar with these topics, as they are indispensable in providing patients with safe and effective spinal deformity correction.

■ Mechanical Properties of Metals

Metals have a common pattern of stress–strain curve consisting of the elastic deformation zone and the plastic deformation zone. In the elastic deformation zone, the stress–strain relationship is linear and the metal deforms in proportion to the applied force (**Fig. 10.1**). After the yield point, the stress–strain curve of metals becomes nonlinear. If increasing force is applied to a metallic implant, the implant will reach the ultimate strength and finally rupture or break.

Table 10.1 History of Metallic Implants Used for Spine Surgery

Year	Event
1890s	Application of sliver wires for spinal fractures
1910s	Development of stainless steel
1920s	Development of cobalt-chromium alloys (Vitallium® in 1932)
1940s	Development of SUS316, 317 stainless steel (Harrington instrumentation)
1960s	Development of titanium alloys (Grade 1–4: commercially pure titanium, other titanium alloys: Ti-6Al-4V, Ti-6Al-7Nb, Ti-6Al-2.5Fe, Ti-13Zr-13Ta, etc.)

Abbreviation: SUS, steel use stainless.

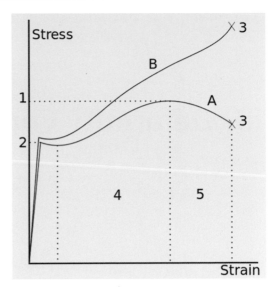

Fig. 10.1 The stress–strain curve of a typical structural metal. Line A shows the apparent stress and line B shows the true stress. Point 1 shows the ultimate strength, and point 2 shows the yield strength. A material demonstrates rupture at point 3. The area of linear relationship between the stress and strain indicates the elastic deformation region before point 2. After point 2, the stress increases up to the ultimate tensile strength (point 1) in region 4. Beyond point 1, a neck forms where the local cross-sectional area significantly decreases and the material becomes weaker in region 5.

Although all metals follow the same pattern of stress–strain relationship, there are differences in their yield strength and ultimate strength and the slope of the stress–strain curve. Within the elastic deformation zone, metals are able to return to the original shape after the force is removed. Once metals were over-bent to their plastic deformation zone, the metal is not able to return to the original shape and permanent deformation of metallic implants occurs. If plastic deformation of the rods occurs after scoliosis correction, significant loss of correction may result, and the original purpose of correcting the spinal deformity would not be fulfilled. For this reason, it is important for spine surgeons to know how much force is put on the spinal implants during correction procedures and mechanical responses of the metallic implants to the forces created by correction procedures.

The metals currently used for spinal deformity surgery include stainless steel, pure titanium, titanium alloys, and Co-Cr alloys. The mechanical properties of each metal are shown in **Fig. 10.2**. Commercial pure titanium (cpTi) has four grades based on its mechanical properties. Grade 1 has the highest value of elongation at break, but it has the lowest tensile strength. As the grade increases, the tensile strength increases, and the capability of elonga-

tion decreases. The tensile strength of Ti alloys is much higher than that of pure titanium, but the elongation capacity of Ti alloys is the lowest among all the types of titanium. Although titanium rods are bent by surgeons during surgery to the desired contour, the mechanical stiffness of titanium decreases significantly around the bending points. Co-Cr shows the highest tensile strength and relatively high break point for elongation. This stiffer mechanical property of Co-Cr is favored by spine surgeons for treatment of rigid spinal deformities. Stainless steel (grade, SUS316L) is a little weaker in its tensile strength compared with Co-Cr, but it shows much better elongation durability. New stainless steel materials with higher tensile strength have been invented recently and will be available for surgery very soon.

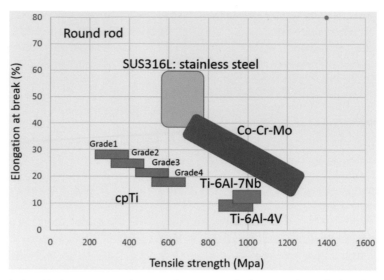

Fig. 10.2 The relationship between tensile strength and elongation at the break of each metal. There are four grades for commercial pure titanium (cpTi), with small differences in mechanical properties. Though titanium alloys show greater tensile strength than cpTi does, the break points of titanium alloys under elongation are much lower than those of cpTi. Stainless steel shows the highest capability for elongation and Co-Cr shows the highest tensile strength among all.

■ Changes in Mechanical Properties of Rods After Manual Bending (Table 10.2)

Because the metallic rods supplied by medical device companies for use during surgery are straight, the surgeon needs to bend them by hand to the desired contour just before performing the correction procedure. With regard to the rods' mechanical properties, the yield strength of titanium alloy rods with a 5.5-mm diameter decreases from 803.9 N to 324.0 N (40.3%) after three-point bending by 20 degrees.[5] The yield strength of titanium alloy rods with a 6.0-mm diameter is reduced 54.1% after 20-degree three-point bending. Co-Cr alloy rods with a 6.0-mm diameter showed the same tendency as the 6.0-mm titanium alloy rods, with their yield significantly decreasing to 56.4% after 20-degree three-point bending. If multiple rod bending operations were performed, even the mechanically stiffest Co-Cr rods can exhibit a significant reduction in their mechanical properties. Spine surgeons should be aware of the reduction in mechanical properties of each metal to avoid mechanical failures of rods

Table 10.2 Changes in Mechanical Properties After Rod Bending[5]

Yield Strength (N)	No Bend	Bend Back One Time	20-Degree Bend	40-Degree Bend
6.0-mm Ti rod	1,004	748 (74.5%)	544 (54.1%)	509 (50.6%)
6.0-mm Co-Cr rod	865	689 (79.6%)	488 (56.4%)	476 (55.0%)
Stiffness (N/mm)				
6.0-mm Ti rod	160	151 (94.6%)	143 (89.2%)	120 (74.9%)
6.0-mm Co-Cr rod	317	278 (87.8%)	261 (82.3%)	208 (65.8%)

Abbreviations: Ti, titanium; Co-Cr, cobalt-chromium.

during surgery and postoperative follow-up periods before solid bony fusion is obtained.

The mechanical forces on spinal implants decrease over time after surgery, as biological bony fusion matures and becomes solid. The maximum force on the spinal implants may occur during the correction procedure. Precise in-vivo forces on spinal implants during correction procedures are still unknown. Previous biomechanical studies have tried to measure in-vivo forces on rods by various engineering methods.[6,7] It is difficult to obtain in-vivo data during operative procedures due to ethical restrictions, and reliable in-vivo data in spinal deformity correction are lacking. Medical devices such as metallic rods and screws for spinal deformity should be designed and manufactured based on the biomechanical and biological environment in which they will be used in the human body. Reliable in-vivo biomechanical information regarding the force on spinal implants during spinal deformity correction may advance the safety and effectiveness of deformity surgery in the future.

■ Viscoelasticity of the Spine

The spinal column, consisting of bone, ligaments, and intervertebral disks, is a composite material with significant viscoelasticity. Viscoelastic materials show two biomechanical characteristics: creep phenomenon and stress relaxation. The creep phenomenon states that when stress is held constant, the strain on the material increases with time. Stress relaxation states that when the strain is held constant, the stress decreases with time.

Considering the viscoelastic property of the spine, rapid correction procedures such as quick rod rotation maneuvers may make the spine much stiffer and may hinder efficient spinal correction, resulting in a lower correction rate than the surgeon anticipated preoperatively. Thus, destabilization procedures, such as bilateral facetectomies, diskectomies, and release of costotransverse ligaments, are very important in obtaining better correction. Besides these technical issues, the biomechanical principles

indicate that slow rod rotation and translation procedures can obtain better final correction rates. After the correction procedure is completed, the rod within an elastic deformation range will tend to spring back to the original shape due to the stress relaxation effect after correction procedures (**Fig. 10.3**). Fast rod rotation may cause significant increase of mechanical loads on the implants and result in dramatic changes in the shape of the rods. If the forces on the rods were within the elastic deformation zone of metal, the rods would still have a potential to return to the original shape. Spine surgeons should be familiar with the mechanical characteristics of metals and the spinal column to obtain better correction rates and provide patients with safe surgery.

■ Correction Procedures for Adolescent Idiopathic Scoliosis

There are many surgical procedures to correct adolescent idiopathic scoliosis (AIS) reported after the introduction of the Harrington instrumentation. The Cobb angle correction on anteroposterior (AP) radiographs was 40% with Harrington rods, 55% with the dual-rod multihook system (CD, Cotrl-Dubousset instrument), and 65% with the dual-rod multiple pedicle screw constructs in the coronal plane. Recent studies reported that pedicle screw constructs in the sagittal plane increased the lordosis of the thoracic spine.[8] While the surgeon is performing the direct vertebral rotation technique to decrease rotational deformity around the apex of the thoracic curve, the major force on the spine pushes the thoracic rib hump down to lessen the rotational deformity of the spine, which eventually causes dekyphosis in the thoracic spine.[9]

There have been several attempts to create thoracic kyphosis by posterior spinal instrumentation surgery. Because a titanium rod is mechanically weaker than a stainless steel or Co-Cr rod, some surgeons utilized stainless steel or Co-Cr rods rather than titanium rods so as

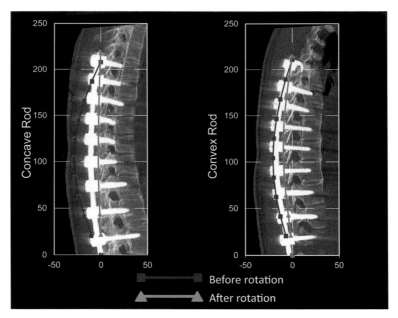

Fig. 10.3 The shape changes of the two rods on both sides of the curve before *(red)* and just after *(blue)* rod rotation and 1 week after surgery *(white)*. The original contours of the two rods showed significant reduction just after the rod rotation procedure. The rods, however, tended to spring back to their original shapes as long as the forces were within the elastic deformation zone of the metal (titanium alloy). The mechanical stress on rods tends to decrease with time due to the stress-relaxation effect of the spine.

not to yield to the force on the rods. Another method was to use an in-situ rod bending technique after a single rod-rotation to create thoracic kyphosis. One of the problems of an in-situ rod-bending procedure is that a much greater load would be applied to the pedicle screws around the area of rod bending, which may increase the possibility of vertebral fractures or screw loosening due to a higher concentration of mechanical force on the screws. Also, multiple rod-bending procedures will reduce the original mechanical strength of the metallic implant.

There have been new surgical techniques for correcting spinal deformity to maintain or create thoracic kyphosis. One technique is the vertebral coplanar alignment (VCA) reported by Vallespir et al.[10] This technique uses slotted tubes attached to each pedicle screw on the convex side of the thoracic curve. Two longitudinal rods are inserted and separated along the slots, driving the tubes into one plane, making the axis of the vertebrae coplanar, thus correct-

ing transverse rotation and coronal translation. For creating thoracic kyphosis, the ends of the tubes are spread in the thoracic spine. After locking a definitive rod on the concave side and retrieving tubes on the concave side, the convex-side rod is inserted and tightened. The curve correction rate in the main thoracic curve was 73% on average, and the average preoperative thoracic kyphosis of 18 degrees remained unchanged after surgery. Another technique is the simultaneous translation technique using two rods as reported by Clement et al.[11] This technique uses polyaxial pedicle screws and polyaxial claws consisting of a pedicle hook and an opposing transverse counter-hook placed at the most cephalad end of the rod. The two 6.0-mm titanium rods are bent first and are inserted pre-oriented. Reduction of the deformity is obtained by gradual and alternate tightening of all nuts on both rods, allowing the vertebrae to gradually approach the rods. Another technique uses a Universal clamp consisting of a woven polyester band, a titanium alloy clamp, and a locking screw as well as pedicle screws.[12] Pedicle screws were placed in two or more vertebrae at the distal extremity of the curve with monaxial screws on the convex side and polyaxial screws on the concave side. Thoracic levels were instrumented with three to seven sublaminar Universal clamps (UCs) on the concave side and one sublaminar UC at the apex on the concave side. Correction of the thoracic curve was performed using posteromedial translation by tightening the UCs for the spine to approach the pre-bent double rods.

The kinematic concept of how to correct the deformity with pedicle screws is shown in **Fig. 10.4**. The apex vertebra should be moved from anterior to posterior and from lateral to medial with two anchor points corresponding to the tips of pedicle screws. The screw tip on the concave side should be moved more posteriorly than that of the convex side. By providing a bigger bend to the concave side rod than to the convex side rod and rotating the two rods simultaneously, the screw tip of the concave side at the apex of the curve moves more posteriorly than that of the convex side does. This technique was reported by Ito et al[13] and named the simultaneous double rod rotation technique, which allows simultaneous correction of the coronal plane deformity and restoration of the thoracic kyphosis. The biomechanically strongest correction procedure, which utilized a solid frame between the pedicle screws on

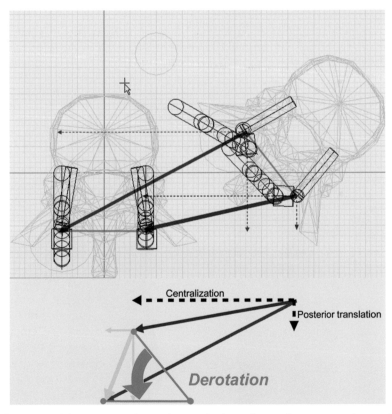

Fig. 10.4 The locations of the apex vertebra in the axial plane. The apex vertebra is located anterolaterally before surgery and the vertebra is to be relocated posteromedially during surgery. The pedicle screw at the apex vertebra on the concave side of the curve should be moved more toward the back *(red line)* than that on the convex side *(blue line)* to relocate the apex vertebra to the normal position. In the simultaneous double rod rotation technique,[13] the concave side rod should be bent more than the convex side rod, which allows the head of the pedicle screw on the concave side to move more toward the back than that on the convex side.

both the convex and concave side of the curve, was reported by Chang and Lenke.[14] By connecting the two rods with a solid metal frame, the spinal implant is able to produce the most powerful force on the spine, but the stress concentration may not occur on specific pedicle screws.

Intraoperative Mechanical Forces on Rods During Rod Rotation Maneuvers

During rod rotation procedures to correct the deformed spine three dimensionally, the inserted rods frequently show dramatic contour changes due to significant mechanical loads on the rods and screws. A recent biomechanical study has used finite element analysis of the mechanical properties of metals and the geometrical changes of metallic rods before and after surgery.[15-17] These authors measured three-dimensional (3D) contour changes of the rods before and after surgery using postoperative 3D computed tomography (CT) images. Specific mathematical assumptions and boundary conditions were put into the computer simulation. In their finite element analysis (FEA) model, the distal end of the rod was fixed completely, and the uppermost end was able to move parallel to the axis of the trunk. By calculating the forces on rods in AIS patients with a single thoracic curve, pullout forces of about 150 N were exerted on the concave side screws around the apex of the curve if pedicle screws were inserted at all the fusion levels (implant density 100%) (**Fig. 10.5**). At both ends of the rods, push-in forces of about 200 N were on the pedicle screws on the concave side of the curve. Push-in forces on pedicle screws rarely result in clinical problems, but pullout forces on screws can lead to screw loosening or bony fractures, which can create serious complications for the

12y.o. F
Lenke 1-A-(-)

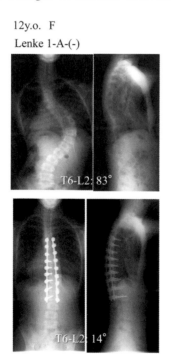

T6-L2: 83°

T6-L2: 14°

Concave side

Rod	curvature		Loss
34.4 degrees	→	18.6 degrees	(−15.7 degrees)

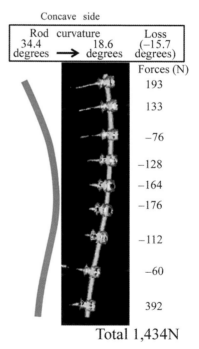

Forces (N)

193

133

−76

−128

−164

−176

−112

−60

392

Total 1,434N

Fig. 10.5 The force on each pedicle screw during rod rotation procedure in an adolescent idiopathic scoliosis (AIS) patient. The contour of the concave side rod shows significant reduction, and pullout forces around the apex of the curve have reached about 200 N according to the calculation. At both ends of the concave side rod, maximum pushing-in force was exerted on the pedicle screws. The minus sign indicates pull-out force on each screw. The total amount of the force acted on the concave side rod has topped 1,400 N.

spinal cord or great vessels. According to the FEA model, the pullout forces on pedicle screws around the apex of the curve may exceed 500 N if the number of pedicle screws were reduced. Maximum pullout forces of thoracic pedicle screws in cadaveric spines are about 600 N, so that there may be an increasing risk of screw pullouts around the apex in patients with rigid curves and fewer pedicle screws.

One of the effective solutions to reduce mechanical forces on pedicle screws is to place cross-links or a frame over the two rods. Many rod rotation procedures utilize only the concave-side rod for correction of scoliosis, and the convex-side rod is placed after completion of rod rotation of the concave side. In these correction procedures, the force on the concave side rod is much higher than that on the convex side rod. The results showed that 50% of the rod contour on the concave side was lost after rod rotation maneuvers and the opposite side rod showed almost no change in its shape. If a cross-link was placed between the two rods, 15% of the total load was shared by the convex side rod, which showed some contour changes. The biomechanically strongest construct with pedicle screws is bilateral screw placement with a cross-link, which forms a triangular shape in each vertebra. From this biomechanical point of view, vertebral column manipulation with a rigid frame cross-linking the two rods and pedicle screws is the most powerful correction procedure in spinal deformity surgery.[14]

Implant Density and Correction Rate

According to the present consensus among spine experts worldwide, AIS curves of less than 70 degrees with flexibility need less than 80% of screw density.[18] From a biomechanical standpoint, a small number of anchors with less rigid metallic rods are not able to correct the spinal deformity sufficiently because they can sustain only small amounts of mechanical load. It seems reasonable to assume that more implant density and more rigid rods will provide better correction rates and final outcomes. Several recent studies, however, found that the final outcome of the surgical correction did not show any significant improvement even if surgeons used more rigid and thicker rods with a higher implant density.[19,20] Implant density and mechanical stiffness of the rods are of some importance to obtain better correction rates. The more important steps to affect the final outcome of deformity correction may be performing preoperative curve flexibility and destabilization procedures, such as Ponte osteotomies, before performing correction procedures including rod rotation and translation.

Chapter Summary

Harrington started to use his spinal implants, consisting of hooks and rods made of stainless steel, for treatment of spinal deformity almost 50 years ago. Since the introduction of his device, surgeries to correct and stabilize the spine with metallic implants have shown dramatic improvement in three-dimensional correction of the curves; an excellent correction rate has been obtained in recent years by using pedicle screws and rigid rods. Titanium alloys are the most popular material for recent spinal surgery due to their biocompatibility and fewer metal-related artifacts on MRI. However, bending a titanium rod multiple times may lead the material to plastic deformation, which makes it significantly weaker mechanically. Surgeons should be familiar with the mechanical characteristics of each material used for deformity surgery and refrain from excessive manual bending of the rods to maintain the original mechanical property of each metal. Spinal implants made of stainless steel or Co-Cr are commonly used for correction of rigid spinal deformities, such as severe scoliosis and rigid kyphosis, because of their superior mechanical stiffness and ability to obtain better correction rates. Surgical treatment of spinal deformity requires familiarity with spinal biomechanics and the mechanical characteristics of each biomaterial. This chapter discussed the fundamentals of biomechanics of spinal deformity correction, mechanical behaviors of metallic implants, in-vivo forces on rods and pedicle screws, biomechanical benefits of destabilization procedures for rigid curves, and viscoelastic properties of the spine. Readers can apply the concepts of spinal biomechanics and material science to their own correction procedures to provide their patients with a safe and effective surgical procedure and excellent clinical outcomes.

Pearls

◆ Spinal deformity correction relies on metallic implants such as screws, hooks, and rods.
◆ Popular metals used for spinal implants are titanium alloys, stainless steel, and cobalt-chromium.

◆ Each metallic material has different mechanical behaviors for the stress–strain relationship and repetitive loading.
◆ The viscoelastic property of the spine should be considered when operating on cases with rigid large spinal deformity.

Pitfalls

◆ Mechanical loads on spinal implants during correction procedures often exceed the limit of bone stiffness, which may lead to surgery-related complications.
◆ Different deformity correction procedures have benefits and limitations.
◆ Rapid rod rotation for rigid deformity correction will significantly increase mechanical loads on the spinal implant.

References.

Five Must-Read References

1. Hadra BE. Wiring of the vertebrae as a means of immobilization in fracture and Pott's disease. The Times and Register, Medical Press, Philadelphia, 1891:1–8
2. Harrington PR. Treatment of scoliosis. Correction and internal fixation by spine instrumentation. J Bone Joint Surg Am 1962;44-A:591–610
3. Suk SI, Lee CK, Kim WJ, Chung YJ, Park YB. Segmental pedicle screw fixation in the treatment of thoracic idiopathic scoliosis. Spine 1995;20:1399–1405
4. Uhthoff HK, Bardos DI, Liskova-Kiar M. The advantages of titanium alloy over stainless steel plates for the internal fixation of fractures. An experimental study in dogs. J Bone Joint Surg Br 1981;63-B:427–484
5. Demura S, Murakami H, Hayashi H, et al. The influence of rod contouring of different spinal constructs on strength and stiffness. Orthopedics, in press
6. Wang X, Aubin CE, Crandall D, Labelle H. Biomechanical modeling and analysis of a direct incremental segmental translation system for the instrumentation of scoliotic deformities. Clin Biomech (Bristol, Avon) 2011;26:548–555
7. Aubin CE, Labelle H, Chevrefils C, Desroches G, Clin J, Eng AB. Preoperative planning simulator for spinal deformity surgeries. Spine 2008;33:2143–2152
8. Sucato DJ, Agrawal S, O'Brien MF, Lowe TG, Richards SB, Lenke L. Restoration of thoracic kyphosis after operative treatment of adolescent idiopathic scoliosis: a multicenter comparison of three surgical approaches. Spine 2008;33:2630–2636
9. Lee SM, Suk SI, Chung ER. Direct vertebral rotation: a new technique of three-dimensional deformity correction with segmental pedicle screw fixation in adolescent idiopathic scoliosis. Spine 2004;29:343–349
10. Vallespir GP, Flores JB, Trigueros IS, et al. Vertebral co-planar alignment: a standardized technique for three dimensional correction in scoliosis surgery: technical description and preliminary results in Lenke type 1 curves. Spine 2008;33:1588–1597
11. Clement JL, Chau E, Geoffray A, Vallade MJ. Simultaneous translation on two rods to treat adolescent idiopathic scoliosis: radiographic results in coronal, sagittal, and transverse plane of a series of 62 patients with a minimum follow-up of two years. Spine 2012;37:184–192
12. Mazda K, Ilharreborde B, Even J, Lefevre Y, Fitoussi F, Pennecot GF. Efficacy and safety of posteromedial translation for correction of thoracic curves in adolescent idiopathic scoliosis using a new connection to the spine: the Universal Clamp. Eur Spine J 2009; 18:158–169
13. Ito M, Abumi K, Kotani Y, et al. Simultaneous double-rod rotation technique in posterior instrumentation surgery for correction of adolescent idiopathic scoliosis. J Neurosurg Spine 2010;12:293–300
14. Chang MS, Lenke LG. Vertebral derotation in adolescent idiopathic scoliosis. Oper Tech Orthop 2009; 19:19–23
15. Salmingo R, Tadano S, Fujisaki K, Abe Y, Ito M. Corrective force analysis for scoliosis from implant rod deformation. Clin Biomech (Bristol, Avon) 2012;27: 545–550

16. Salmingo RA, Tadano S, Fujisaki K, Abe Y, Ito M. Relationship of forces acting on implant rods and degree of scoliosis correction. Clin Biomech (Bristol, Avon) 2013;28:122–128

17. Salmingo RA, Tadano S, Abe Y, Ito M. Influence of implant rod curvature on sagittal correction of scoliosis deformity. Spine J 2014;14:1432–1439

18. de Kleuver M, Lewis SJ, Germscheid NM, et al. Optimal surgical care for adolescent idiopathic scoliosis: an international consensus. Eur Spine J 2014;23: 2603–2618

19. Prince DE, Matsumoto H, Chan CM, et al. The effect of rod diameter on correction of adolescent idiopathic scoliosis at two years follow-up. J Pediatr Orthop 2014;34:22–28

20. Chen J, Yang C, Ran B, et al. Correction of Lenke 5 adolescent idiopathic scoliosis using pedicle screw instrumentation: does implant density influence the correction? Spine 2013;38:E946–E951

11

Pseudarthrosis and Infection

Michael P. Kelly and Sigurd Berven

■ Introduction

Adult spinal deformity (ASD) is among the most challenging pathologies treated by spine surgeons. Preoperative preparation to correct neural element compression as well as coronal and sagittal malalignment requires strict attention to detail and near-perfect technical execution. Surgery to treat ASD can be frustrating, however, as a seemingly "perfect" surgery may still be complicated in the both near- and long-term periods by complications requiring unanticipated revision surgery. Two such common complications are pseudarthrosis and infection. Our group has reported a 9% rate of unanticipated second procedures in adults undergoing primary surgery for ASD, where pseudarthrosis (4%) and infection (1%) were common causes for revision.[1] Even more troublesome was a 21% rate of repeat revision surgery, where pseudarthrosis (5%) and infection (2%) were again two common causes.[2] These numbers are in line with reports from other cohorts; thus, pseudarthrosis remains a common cause of revision surgery in primary and revision ASD.[3,4]

■ Pseudarthrosis

Successful fusion requires optimal biological and biomechanical environments, which rely on both patient selection and surgical technique.

Although advances in implant technology and osteobiologics have improved union rates, pseudarthroses persist in as many as 16% of three-column osteotomy patients.[5,6] This is a result of the risk factors for pseudarthrosis that exist by the nature of ASD surgeries. Long-segment fusions are at a higher risk for pseudarthrosis because of the large surface area of bone that must heal. In addition, the commonly employed midline approach is associated with a denervation of the paraspinal musculature, with an associated decrease in vascularity to this musculature. This is an insult to the local healing environment. ASD surgeries are not uncommonly associated with spinal stenosis, requiring decompression, or rigid coronal and sagittal plane deformities, requiring posterior column osteotomies. The greater the amount of bone resected, the greater the theoretical risk of a pseudarthrosis developing. Despite modern implants, a long segment fusion will remain somewhat mobile, through elastic deformation of the construct. This micromotion, in some cases, may be excessive, without the rigidity required to promote fusion. In the absence of a fusion mass, implants will almost certainly fracture. This may occur as early as 6 months to 1 year, though we have encountered pseudarthrosis that presented a late as 7 years postoperatively (**Fig. 11.1**). Finally, ASD often involves fusion of junctional segments (e.g., lumbosacral junction, thoracolumbar junction), which are at a higher risk of nonunion.[6] In some cases, ante-

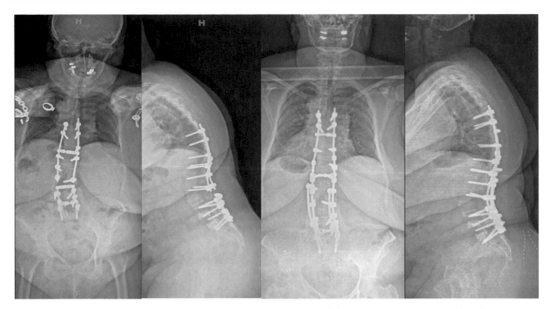

Fig. 11.1 A 50-year-old woman presented 8 years after L3 pedicle subtraction osteotomy with broken implants and pseudarthrosis causing fixed sagittal plane malalignment. She was treated with revision posterior spinal fusion; note the four rods spanning the level of the pedicle subtraction.

rior column support, through either a transforaminal lumbar interbody fusion (TLIF) or an anterior lumbar interbody fusion (ALIF), may assist with improving union rates. Appropriate use of recombinant human bone morphogenetic protein-2 (rh-BMP2) at the lumbosacral junction may obviate the use of TLIF/ALIF at L5-S1.

Nicotine exposure is associated with decreased fusion rates in spine surgery. In the case of ASD, the risk of nonunion with multilevel surgery is great and, in our practice, surgery is not offered to patients who are unable to cease nicotine use. To test for nicotine use, we routinely check urine cotinine levels. This metabolite of nicotine is excreted in the urine and offers reliable values for active and passive exposure to cigarette smoke, making it a suitable screening test for this patient population. Nicotine has proven antiangiogenic effects on fusion masses, increasing the likelihood of nonunion. Furthermore, nicotine has been shown to have an adverse influence on patient-reported outcomes in several areas of spine surgery, independent of other risk factors, further decreasing the potential for success with surgery.

Given the costs and risks associated with spinal deformity surgery, nicotine cessation is necessary. In most cases, we require 3 months of preoperative abstinence, to prove that the cessation is lasting.

Osteoporosis is increasingly common in ASD patients, as the age of patients seeking surgery rises. Perhaps even more common is hypovitaminosis D, which has been shown to be common in general orthopedic surgery practices and in spine surgery–specific practices.[7] Vitamin D plays an essential role in bone metabolism and homeostasis, and low vitamin D levels are associated with osteomalacia (hypomineralized bone). We routinely check serum 25-hydroxyvitamin D levels at preoperative visits, and we prescribe supplementation with oral vitamin D as needed. In most cases, 50,000 International Units (IU) weekly for 6 weeks, followed by 1,000 IU daily. In addition, we recommend supplementation with 1,000 mg of calcium daily. In some cases, hypovitaminosis D exists due to some other systemic pathology, rather than malnutrition. For these patients, we consult endocrinologists with a particular interest in bone metabolism.

As previously mentioned, however, osteoporosis is a common comorbidity encountered by spine surgeons. This is of concern to surgeons, as bone mineral density (BMD) is directly correlated with insertional torque and pullout strength. Strength of screw purchase, in turn, affects fusion rates by determining the durability and rigidity of the construct and its stability while the fusion mass matures. We routinely obtain bone densitometry tests such as dual-energy X-ray absorptiometry (DEXA) scans preoperatively. These tests provide the true value of the BMD and the T-score, which is the number of standard deviations above or below the mean for young-adult reference standards. Osteoporosis is defined as a T-score of –2.5 or lower. Osteopenia exists at between –1 and –2.5 standard deviations. When ordering a DEXA scan, one must remember that in many cases the lumbar spine BMD may be falsely elevated due to spondylosis, with endplate sclerosis and osteophyte formation (**Fig. 11.2**). The DEXA scan should include densities at the hip and distal radius. We have found the distal radius particularly useful for making the diagnosis of osteoporosis, which facilitates pharmacological management of the disorder.

Although a multitude of options exist for the management of osteoporosis, only one anabolic therapy exists, teriparatide (Forteo, Eli Lilly, Indianapolis, IN).[8] Teriparatide is a recombinant form of a portion of the parathyroid hormone (PTH). Although PTH increases osteoclastic activity, via osteoblast signaling, pulsatile administration of teriparatide increases osteoblastic activity to a greater degree, increasing bone formation. An adverse effect of teriparatide observed in animal models was osteosarcoma formation, however, and patients with risk factors for osteosarcoma, including Paget's disease and prior radiation therapy, should avoid teriparatide exposure. In cases of a contraindication to teriparatide, we often employ denosumab, a monoclonal antibody that binds receptor activator of nuclear-κB (RANK) ligand (RANKL). The binding of RANKL prevents RANK activations, thereby suppressing osteoclast activation. This is an "anti-catabolic" mechanism of osteoporosis management, however, similar to bisphosphonates. Both denosumab and bisphosphonates delay callus maturation in fracture models, which likely behave similarly to a fusion model, but there is no human evidence to support a correlation between exposure to these anti-catabolic medications and pseudarthrosis.[8] Nonetheless, we attempt to avoid bisphosphonate exposure early in the spine fusion process, as there are animal data to support a negative effect of bisphosphonates. There is some evidence, however, that a combination of teriparatide and bisphosphonate therapy may be ideal to maximize callus formation and rigidity, with early teriparatide administration followed by conversion to bisphosphonate therapy.

Surgical techniques may play a role in instrumenting the osteoporotic spine as well. Specially designed screw threads have been shown to increase insertional torque, which may benefit the durability of a construct in osteoporotic bone. Hydroxyapatite coating has also been shown to increase screw purchase. As the pedicle is often patulous in the osteoporotic spine, one may choose to avoid tapping the channel of the pedicle screw. If tapping is per-

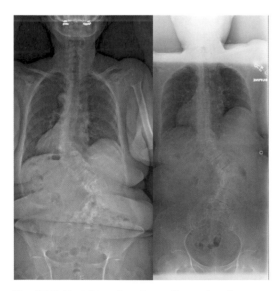

Fig. 11.2 Upright and supine radiographs of a 65-year-old woman with degenerative lumbar scoliosis. Note the hypertrophic osteoarthritis through the apex of the deformity, which would cause a falsely elevated bone mineral density.

formed, it should undersize the anticipated screw diameter by 1 mm or more. Screw diameters should be maximized, at least 70% of pedicle diameter, to ensure an appropriate interference fit within the pedicle. Screw length should be maximized and, in extreme cases, one may choose to tap the anterior cortex and achieve bicortical purchase of the screw, as this will significantly improve pullout strength. One should attempt to leave the dorsal cortex intact as well, as this may minimize screw toggling and loosening.

Implant materials are a matter of preference and are debated among spinal deformity surgeons. We prefer to use 5.5-mm cobalt-chromium (Co-Cr) rods in cases of degenerative scoliosis with poor bone quality. In larger, stiffer reconstructions, we commonly use a 6.0-mm Co-Cr rod on the "working side," and place a 5.5-mm Co-Cr on the contralateral side. Some surgeons prefer commercially pure titanium rods, which are a bit less stiff than Co-Cr, believing that this will stress the bone–implant interface less, thereby decreasing the incidence of adjacent segment problems. Conversely, some surgeons prefer 6.35-mm stainless steel (SS) rods, believing this is the most durable metal for spinal deformity surgery. In a series of spinal deformity patients, implant fracture was less common among those fixed with Co-Cr rods.[9] In cases of three-column osteotomy (i.e., pedicle subtraction osteotomy, vertebral column resection), dominoes are used to span the osteotomy level with more than two rods, increasing the rigidity of the construct at the osteotomy site and decreasing micromotion. In any case, secure fixation, with accurate screw placement, is required along the length of the deformity. This increases the rigidity of the construct, decreasing nonunion rates. We perform high-density instrumentation (1.8 screws/level) in the vast majority of ASD surgeries. Although this issue is debated regarding adolescent idiopathic scoliosis, we feel strongly that high-density instrumentation is needed in ASD.

In all cases instrumented to S1, we place distal supporting screws, often S2-alar-iliac (S2AI) or iliac screws.[10] Iliac screws distal to S1 decrease strain on S1 fixation in flexion, minimizing micromotion at the lumbosacral junction. S2AI screws have been proposed as an alternative to iliac screws, with a more ventral starting point and "in-line" tulip heads, facilitating rod placement. Midterm results of S2AI screws are encouraging, and we employ this technique frequently. A third option for distal fixation is S2-alar screws. These screws offer support to S1 pullout, without crossing or immobilizing the sacroiliac joint. If one chooses to use this method, attention must be paid to the course of the L5 root, as it courses over the front of the sacral ala. Bone graft materials should consist of locally obtained autograft, allograft, and iliac crest bone graft (ICBG) or rbBMP-2. We routinely use fresh-frozen cancellous allograft, as its osteoinductive properties are likely better than those of cortical chips. In long fusions, inadequate volumes of ICBG may indicate the use of rh-BMP2 in an off-label fashion. We have shown this to be an effective method of improving fusion rates. We neither use nor advocate other so-called osteobiologic products, as the evidence to support their use is weak. The dorsal elements should be decorticated, using gauges or burs, to fresh bleeding bone. Bleeding bone is a requisite for competitive fusion rates. If using more than two rods or cross-links, they are fixed after bone graft placement, to minimize disruption and interference with contiguous grafting.

In the vast majority of cases, the diagnosis of pseudarthrosis is made with the presence of loose or fractured implants. We intervene when there is a progression of deformity or pain. In the absence of progression, we often observe unilateral rod fractures. When both rods have fractured, we usually recommend revision surgery. In a small number of cases, a pseudarthrosis may present as symptoms consistent with neural element compression (e.g., radiculopathy, claudication) due to scar tissue/fibrous callus accumulation (**Fig. 11.3**). Computed tomography (CT), with fine cuts and metal subtraction, is the preferred imaging modality for diagnosing pseudarthrosis.[11] Flexion/extension radiographs have been used, though they are not as sensitive as CT scanning.

Management of pseudarthrosis consists of revision surgery. The use of rh-BMP2 in posterolateral fusion revisions has received Food

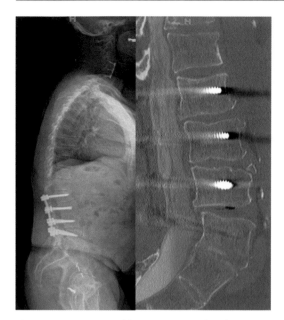

Fig. 11.3 A 61-year-old man presented with a sagittal plane malalignment and L4 radiculopathy due to pseudarthrosis. Note the vacuum disk within the instrumented levels, indicative of a pseudarthrosis.

and Drug Administration (FDA) approval. When revising a pseudarthrosis case, inspection of the entire fusion mass is recommended, as one pseudarthrosis may beget another.[12] In our experience, most pseudarthrosis presents at L5-S1, L4-L5, and at the thoracolumbar junction, in that order. Revision surgery often consists of anterior column support, if not already done, in the form of a TLIF, ALIF, or transpsoas interbody fusion. Options for graft material include titanium, polyetheretherketone (PEEK), and allograft. Our preference is to use titanium, as it bonds to bone, increasing the stability of the construct and likely improving fusion rates. The pseudarthrosis tissue should be debrided, as these tissues are unable to undergo mineralization and must be removed to achieve union. In the lumbar spine, we often perform a posterior column osteotomy through the pseudarthrosis tissue and compress through the pseudarthrosis. In addition to encouraging fusion by exposure of bleeding cancellous bone, the osteotomy aids in restoration of lordosis, taking tension off of the fusion mass and promoting compression at

the pseudarthrosis level. If rh-BMP2 is not used, we use autogenous iliac crest graft, as the biologic activity of allograft is not sufficient to create a competitive environment for fusion in the setting of a previous pseudarthrosis. For cases of lumbosacral junction pseudarthrosis, we ensure that we have adequate distal fixation, consisting of pedicle screws at the first sacral vertebra and iliac screws below that. In the case of patulous, eroded S1 pedicles, we place multiple iliac screws on each side.

The postoperative routine is unchanged in the management of pseudarthrosis. No bracing is used and the patients are mobilized on postoperative day 1. Strict activity precautions are established, however, and patients are instructed on how to safely rise from bed and are given a front-wheeled walker to use for 6 weeks to encourage an upright posture, discouraging flexion through the revision fusion mass. Teriparatide therapy is continued for a minimum of 3 months after surgery. We do not perform CT scanning for evaluation of fusion masses, as the exposure to radiation is excessive, and findings are unlikely to affect our management of the patient.

Careful attention to detail in preoperative planning, intraoperative performance, and postoperative rehabilitation helps surgeons minimize pseudarthrosis in their practice. Smoking cessation is absolutely mandatory to ensure competitive results. Appropriate choices of biologics and instrumentation help increase fusion rates. However, a nonunion rate of 0% is not realistic, and the informed decision-making process should include discussion of the risk of reoperation for nonunion in ASD surgery.

■ Infection

Perioperative surgical-site infection (SSI) is a significant cause of morbidity in ASD surgery, with reported rates ranging from 0.3% to 20%.[1,2,13] These rates include both superficial and deep wound infections; the treatments and implications for each differ. In many instances, a superficial infection can be managed on an outpatient basis, with oral antibiotics alone.

Conversely, a deep wound infection is a catastrophe, nearly universally managed with rehospitalization, revision surgery, and prolonged intravenous antibiotics followed by oral antibiotics.

A review of the Scoliosis Research Society (SRS) Morbidity and Mortality database revealed an overall infection rate of 2.1% in cases performed by participating members.[13] This cohort included a heterogeneous mix of procedures, including noninstrumented degenerative lumbar surgeries, in addition to instrumented ASD procedures. Not surprisingly, less extensive surgeries, including lumbar diskectomies and minimally invasive TLIF procedures were associated with lower rates of infection. Those cases that were associated with instrumented spinal fusions had higher rates of infection. Neuromuscular scoliosis (14%) and postlaminectomy kyphosis (5.1%) had the highest rates of postoperative wound infection. Revision surgeries were more commonly affected by infections (3.3% vs 2.0%), and deep infections were more common in this situation as well.

Although the SRS database provides good epidemiological data regarding rates of infections, it does not provide the granular data that allow for finer conclusions regarding postoperative infections in the ASD population. Several smaller series have reviewed the rates of reoperation for patients undergoing ASD reconstructions. Pichelmann et al[1] published our group's experience with primary ASD surgeries, noting a rate of reoperation for infection of 1.4% and accounting for 15.5% of revision surgeries. One must note that this rate is likely lower than the true value, as superficial infections are unlikely to have undergone reoperation. As a follow-up study, we reviewed the rates of unanticipated reoperation for revision ASD procedures, noting infection in 14% of revision surgeries performed.[2] These rates are similar to those presented by others, with infection accounting for 15% of revision surgeries in ASD.[3]

Adult spinal deformity surgeries are at higher risk for perioperative infection than other orthopedic or neurologic surgeries because of the long duration, high estimated blood losses, large surface areas, and extensive use of implants. It stands to reason that the longer a wound is exposed to air, the more likely some contamination may occur. High estimated blood losses are often associated with the need for perioperative allogeneic transfusions. Although allogeneic transfusions are associated with major complications, such as transfusion-related acute lung injury (TRALI), more common are perioperative infections, including SSI, urinary tract infections, and respiratory tract infections.[14] The exposure to allogeneic blood and proteins is associated with an immunomodulatory effect that may depress the immune response to pathogens, making the patient susceptible to SSI. This relationship has been shown in less extensive lumbar degenerative fusion procedures and the same is likely true in ASD.

Implants render patients susceptible to deep wound infections, as there is a race between native cells and bacteria to the implant surface. Bacteria form a glycocalyx on implants, which helps them adhere to the surface. The glycocalyx "protects" the bacteria from antibiotics, due to poor penetrance by antibiotics, and also decreases the value of wound culture, as bacteria become adherent to the glycocalyx and are not easily shed into the wound bed. There is evidence that titanium and cobalt chromium implants are less susceptible to glycocalyx formation than stainless steel. Our preference is to use Co-Cr rods for their material properties in ASD.

Patient demographics certainly help identify those at risk for developing SSI. Thus, as with pseudarthrosis, it is imperative that these patients are identified and that appropriate steps are taken to minimize the risk of SSI. A comprehensive review of patients treated at our institution, with an overall deep infection rate of 2.0%, found that a concomitant diagnosis of diabetes had the strongest association with a perioperative infection (odds ratio [OR], 3.5).[15] The importance of controlled blood glucose levels was emphasized, as even patients without a diagnosis of diabetes but with episodes of hyperglycemia showed a higher rate of infection. These findings were later supported by Richards et al,[16] who found an increased rate of infection in orthopedic trauma patients with poorly controlled perioperative blood glucose levels. Obesity (body mass index 30–35 kg/m^2) was also associated with an increased risk of infection (OR, 2/2).

Preincision antibiotic prophylaxis is mandatory, and antibiotics must be given at the appropriate time. We have shown a 3.4-fold increased risk of infection in those patients who did not receive intravenous cefazolin within 1 hour of incision. In a study of pediatric spinal deformity surgeries, Milstone et al[17] found a similar relationship between infections and inappropriate antibiotic administration timing. The choice of prophylactic antibiotics may vary by institution, but it should consist of an antibiotic with broad-spectrum gram-positive coverage of common skin flora. At our institution, prophylaxis is provided with cefazolin and vancomycin. In the case of penicillin or cephalosporin allergy, we use aztreonam. Both antibiotics are given within 1 hour of the skin incision, with vancomycin started earlier to provide an appropriate rate of administration and to minimize the risk of red man syndrome. During surgery, we re-dose antibiotics at half the time of normal administration. For example, cefazolin is given every 4 hours, as it is normally given every 8 hours.

Intra-site antibiotics, commonly in the form of lyophilized vancomycin powder, administered at the time of wound closure are becoming increasingly common. Several retrospective analyses have shown decreased rates of SSI with the institution of this technique. Sweet et al[18] published the first report on this method, noting a decreased prevalence from 2.6% to 0.2% with the use of intra-site vancomycin in adult spine patients. This benefit has been supported by several other studies in adult and pediatric spine surgeries. There have been no complications definitively linked to the use of intra-site vancomycin powder, though there are concerns about pseudarthrosis, anaphylaxis, and "super-infection." Vancomycin is acidic and changes the environment within the wound bed, though no effect on union rates has been observed. Vancomycin powder is effective in eliminating gram-positive contaminants, but some concern over an increase in gram-negative and polymicrobial infections exists. A single randomized controlled trial did not support the effectiveness of lyophilized vancomycin powder.[19] Nonetheless, our experience mirrors those of others, and we continue to employ this practice.

We place both superficial and deep drains at the time of wound closure. There is limited but not strong evidence supporting their use in spinal deformity surgery. Blank et al[20] performed a randomized trial of surgical drains in patients undergoing surgery for adolescent idiopathic scoliosis. They found increased rates of wound drainage in those patients treated without a drain. The study was underpowered and thus could not detect a difference in infection rates, however. It stands to reason that an adequately powered study would support a decreased rate of postoperative infection with decreased wound drainage. Postoperative drains have been associated with increased rates of perioperative blood transfusions, and this must be balanced with the potential benefit of wound drainage.

Diagnosis of spine infections can often be made with a history and physical examination. Fevers and chills as well as lethargy/malaise are common—the former are more frequent with acute infections, and the latter are more common with chronic, deep infections. In the case of acute infections, some may show wound erythema, fluctuance, and wound drainage. These signs are not ubiquitous, however, and the clinician must have some level of suspicion. In chronic infections, a small draining sinus is common, or a new and enlarging fluctuant mass may be present. Upon presentation, one should draw a complete blood count and serum C-reactive protein (CRP). We have found CRP to be more useful than the erythrocyte sedimentation rate (ESR) in diagnosing postoperative infections. In the immediate postoperative period, the half-life of CRP is ~ 2.5 days, whereas the kinetics of ESR are of little utility. Imaging of the spine should begin with plain radiographs, which may show evidence of screw loosening, with halos, in cases of chronic infection (**Fig. 11.4**). Following plain radiographs, CT or magnetic resonance imaging are of limited utility, as a seroma forms in all cases, regardless of bacterial contamination. Aspiration

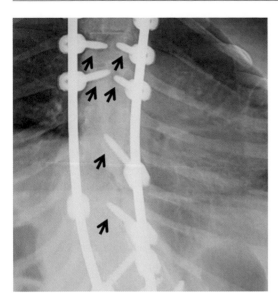

Fig. 11.4 An 11-year-old girl with neuromuscular scoliosis presented with pain 11 months after posterior spinal fusion. Exploration revealed a deep wound infection. Note the lucencies *(arrows)* surrounding the midthoracic pedicle screws.

of a seroma and fluid analysis may be performed when there is uncertainty regarding the presence of an infection. Physician suspicion and concern should drive the decision to intervene for a suspected infection.

Management of a superficial infection is often successful with antibiotics alone, as this is usually a cellulitis related to the surgical wound. Acute, deep wound infections are treated aggressively in our practice. The standard of care is irrigation and debridement. In the wound is grossly contaminated, we may remove loose graft. In the absence of gross contamination, graft and implants are retained. Effort should be made to achieve good decontamination of the wound, so that implants can be retained. Although their presence as a foreign body might concern surgeons, the instability caused by implant removal will make eradication of the infection more difficult. If there is any question regarding the level of contamination of the wound, we place a wound vacuum-assisted closure (WVAC) dressing and return to the operating room in 72 hours for repeat irrigation and debridement, with possible WVAC change

versus delayed primary closure. A chronic, delayed deep wound infection is treated differently, however. These infections are more commonly associated with less virulent bacteria, such as *Propionibacterium acnes* or *Staphylococcus epidermidis*. As these bacteria are less virulent, and grow more slowly, intraoperative cultures should be taken and incubated for a longer period than normal, 14 to 28 days. In cases of chronic, delayed infection, we remove implants and confirm the arthrodesis and the absence of pseudarthrosis. Patients are followed for evidence of curve progression or pseudarthrosis in follow-up and are re-instrumented only when needed for deformity progression.

When successfully treated, patients with deep wound infection following ASD surgery can expect good outcomes, equivalent to those of patients who did not encounter this complication.[21]

■ Chapter Summary

Pseudarthrosis and infection are two common reasons for revision surgery in adult spinal deformity. Both of these pathologies have risk factors that are modifiable by both the patient and the surgeon. Nicotine avoidance is mandatory in ASD, given the already high rate of perioperative complications associated with these surgeries. Evaluation of bone health, with bone mineral density testing, and treatment of osteoporosis should be routine. Appropriate management of diabetes mellitus, including tight control of perioperative blood glucose levels, will help minimize risks of perioperative infection. Antibiotic prophylaxis should be given within an hour of incision and be tailored to prophylaxis against common flora in the community.

As techniques evolve, with concomitant improvements in implants and biologic therapies, the rates of these two complications will fall. Ultimately, meticulous attention to detail before, during, and after surgery will maximize the likelihood of success and minimize complications in these patients.

Pearls

- Smoking cessation is necessary in adult spinal deformity surgery.
- Evaluation for osteoporosis, with bone mineral density testing, and appropriate pharmacological intervention should be performed in ASD patients.
- Teriparatide is an anabolic agent available for management of osteoporosis and may have some benefit in achieving arthrodesis.
- Facetectomies must be performed, and decortication of dorsal elements is necessary.
- Recombinant human bone morphogenetic protein-2 decreases rates of reoperation for pseudarthrosis in ASD.
- Informed consent specifically tailored to the use of rh-BMP2 in both on-label and off-label applications (addressing risks of pain, seroma, ectopic bone, and potential for malignancy) should be sought from the patient.
- Iliac or S2-alar-iliac screws should be placed routinely, when fusing to S1.
- High-density (≥ 1.8 screws/level) constructs are recommended in ASD.
- Patient factors associated with surgical-site infections in ASD include high body mass index and poorly controlled diabetes mellitus.
- Prophylactic, intravenous antibiotics must be administered within 1 hour of incision.

- Prophylactic, intra-site, lyophilized vancomycin powder may decrease rates of surgical-site infection.
- Aggressive management of acute, deep wound infections offers patients a chance for equivalent outcomes once the complication has resolved.

Pitfalls

- Nicotine exposure increases rates of pseudarthrosis. One must resist the desire to operate on patients who are using nicotine products and insist that they be compliant with smoking cessation prior to surgery.
- Implants and osteobiologics do not compensate for poor planning and execution of technique in ASD. Poor planning and performance increase rates of pseudarthrosis and surgical-site infection.
- The use of rh-BMP2 without informed consent from the patient is ill-advised.
- Inadequate debridement of pseudarthrosis tissue increases the likelihood of recurrent pseudarthrosis.
- Prophylactic antibiotics must be administered within 1 hour of incision. Cefazolin should be given every 4 hours during surgery.
- Poorly controlled postoperative blood glucose levels increase the risk of infection.

References
Five Must-Read References

1. Pichelmann MA, Lenke LG, Bridwell KH, Good CR, O'Leary PT, Sides BA. Revision rates following primary adult spinal deformity surgery: six hundred forty-three consecutive patients followed-up to twenty-two years postoperative. Spine 2010;35:219–226

2. Kelly MP, Lenke LG, Bridwell KH, Agarwal R, Godzik J, Koester L. Fate of the adult revision spinal deformity patient: a single institution experience. Spine 2013;38:E1196–E1200

3. Richards M. Unanticipated revision surgery in adult spinal deformity: an experience with 815 cases at one institution. Spine 2014;39(26, Suppl 1):S174–182

4. Mok JM, Cloyd JM, Bradford DS, et al. Reoperation after primary fusion for adult spinal deformity: rate, reason, and timing. Spine 2009;34:832–839

5. Kim HJ, Buchowski JM, Zebala LP, Dickson DD, Koester L, Bridwell KH. RhBMP-2 is superior to iliac crest bone graft for long fusions to the sacrum in adult spinal deformity: 4- to 14-year follow-up. Spine 2013;38:1209–1215

6. Kim YJ, Bridwell KH, Lenke LG, Rhim S, Cheh G. Pseudarthrosis in long adult spinal deformity instrumentation and fusion to the sacrum: prevalence and risk factor analysis of 144 cases. Spine 2006;31:2329–2336

7. Stoker GE, Buchowski JM, Bridwell KH, Lenke LG, Riew KD, Zebala LP. Preoperative vitamin D status of adults undergoing surgical spinal fusion. Spine 2013;38:507–515

8. Hirsch BP, Unnanuntana A, Cunningham ME, Lane JM. The effect of therapies for osteoporosis on spine fusion: a systematic review. Spine J 2013;13:190–199

9. Smith JS, Shaffrey CI, Ames CP, et al; International Spine Study Group. Assessment of symptomatic rod fracture after posterior instrumented fusion for adult spinal deformity. Neurosurgery 2012;71:862–867

10. Kebaish KM. Sacropelvic fixation: techniques and complications. Spine 2010;35:2245–2251

11. Carreon LY, Djurasovic M, Glassman SD, Sailer P. Diagnostic accuracy and reliability of fine-cut CT scans

with reconstructions to determine the status of an instrumented posterolateral fusion with surgical exploration as reference standard. Spine 2007;32:892–895

12. Pateder DB, Park YS, Kebaish KM, et al. Spinal fusion after revision surgery for pseudarthrosis in adult scoliosis. Spine 2006;31:E314–E319

13. Smith JS, Shaffrey CI, Sansur CA, et al; Scoliosis Research Society Morbidity and Mortality Committee. Rates of infection after spine surgery based on 108,419 procedures: a report from the Scoliosis Research Society Morbidity and Mortality Committee. Spine 2011;36:556–563

14. Woods BI, Rosario BL, Chen A, et al. The association between perioperative allogeneic transfusion volume and postoperative infection in patients following lumbar spine surgery. J Bone Joint Surg Am 2013;95: 2105–2110

15. Olsen MA, Nepple JJ, Riew KD, et al. Risk factors for surgical site infection following orthopaedic spinal operations. J Bone Joint Surg Am 2008;90:62–69

16. Richards JE, Kauffmann RM, Zuckerman SL, Obremskey WT, May AK. Relationship of hyperglycemia and surgical-site infection in orthopaedic surgery. J Bone Joint Surg Am 2012;94:1181–1186

17. Milstone AM, Maragakis LL, Townsend T, et al. Timing of preoperative antibiotic prophylaxis: a modifiable risk factor for deep surgical site infections after pediatric spinal fusion. Pediatr Infect Dis J 2008;27:704–708

18. Sweet FA, Roh M, Sliva C. Intrawound application of vancomycin for prophylaxis in instrumented thoracolumbar fusions: efficacy, drug levels, and patient outcomes. Spine 2011;36:2084–2088

19. Tubaki VR, Rajasekaran S, Shetty AP. Effects of using intravenous antibiotic only versus local intrawound vancomycin antibiotic powder application in addition to intravenous antibiotics on postoperative infection in spine surgery in 907 patients. Spine 2013; 38:2149–2155

20. Blank J, Flynn JM, Bronson W. The use of postoperative subcutaneous closed suction drainage after posterior spinal fusion in adolescents with idiopathic scoliosis. J Spinal Disord Tech 2003;16(6):508–512

21. Mok JM, Guillaume TJ, Talu U, et al. Clinical outcome of deep wound infection after instrumented posterior spinal fusion: a matched cohort analysis. Spine 2009;34:578–583

Index

Note: Page references followed by *f* or *t* indicate pages or tables, respectively.